Winning

the
Weight Loss War

How I Lost 100 Pounds for Good

- and How You Can, Too.

RIVKA   FUCHS

Winning the Weight Loss War

How I Lost 100 Pounds for Good

– and How You Can, Too.

Copyright © 2015 by Rivka Fuchs

For permission requests or to contact the author,

please email:

rivkafuchscoach@gmail.com

ISBN 978-0-9969587-0-7

Printed in the United States of America

Table of Contents

Introduction   1

Chapter ~ 1 ~
  Let's Start at the Beginning
  ~ My Story to Help You Write Your Own Story ~   3
Chapter ~ 1 ~
  "Write Your Own Story"   9

Chapter ~ 2 ~
  Mistakes I Made Along the Way
  ~ What Kept Me in Yo-Yo Mode for More
        than Forty Years ~   11
Chapter ~ 2 ~
  "Write Your Own Story"   15

Chapter ~ 3 ~
  What I Did to Lose Weight
  ~ Strategies that Worked ~   17
Chapter ~ 3 ~
  "Write Your Own Story"   37

Chapter ~ 4 ~
  Audio Messages
  ~ Positive Thoughts & the Art of Relaxation ~   39
Chapter ~ 4 ~
  "Write Your Own Story"   51

Chapter ~ 5 ~
  Cognitive Changes for Success
  ~ The Mind is a Powerful Aid ~   53
Chapter ~ 5 ~
  "Write Your Own Story"   68

Chapter ~ 6 ~
Dealing with Hunger
~ Strategies to Overcome Hunger ~   71
Chapter ~ 6 ~
"Write Your Own Story"   80

Chapter ~ 7 ~
Spirituality
~ Embracing G-d's Help ~   83
Chapter ~ 7 ~
"Write Your Own Story"   90

Chapter ~ 8 ~
Food Changes for Success
~ Quality of Food Does Matter ~   93
Chapter ~ 8 ~
"Write Your Own Story"   112

Chapter ~ 9 ~
Maintenance
~ Think, Eat, Drink and Stay Slim ~   115
Chapter ~ 9 ~
"Write Your Own Story"   122

Chapter ~ 10 ~
Time to Write Your Own Story
~ Compilation of End-of-Chapter Notes ~   125
Chapter ~ 10 ~
"Write Your Own Story"   129

About the Author   133

Acknowledgments   135

Introduction

My weight loss journey began in childhood and finally resulted in losing over 100 pounds that I have kept off naturally for more than twenty years. No surgery and no diet pills. Just healthy habits and a solid commitment to reach my goal.

This book is my weight loss story. It is an accumulation of more than 20 years of trial and error in the weight loss war.

Everyone needs a personal weight loss plan to be successful. One size does not fit all. But, the one universal thing we all need for lasting results is a holistic approach – one that focuses not only on the body, but the mind and soul as well. This was my biggest discovery; that the way to true weight loss was so much more than counting calories, simple tips and tricks, or harnessing my "willpower." It was addressing deeper thoughts and emotions.

To that end, the workbook format in this book is to help you write your own story. At the end of every chapter there is a "Write Your Own Story" section with questions and blank pages for you to write down your answers. These questions are to help you determine what will best aid you in your efforts to lose weight. Not only do they inquire as to your current eating habits, they also take a look at what is beyond the food on your plate.

I knew that I had to look inward, and that there were questions to answer. How has being overweight impacted your life? Are you always seeking answers from others? Are you ready to trust yourself? Do you know what works for you and what does not? What do you need in your plan to fit your lifestyle? What are your triggers? These are the kinds of questions that play into your weight loss challenge.

For a long time, my discoveries were only benefitting *me*. Even for those who approached me wanting to know how "I did it," my advice never captured the full picture. I wanted to help more.

So I went back to school. I became a Certified Life Coach, Master Coach & Counselor, and Integrative Nutrition Health Coach. By combining methodologies from all my training with my personal experience, I am able to help clients reach their health goals in a realistic, sustainable way.

Chapter
~ 1 ~

Let's Start at the Beginning

~ My Story to Help You Write Your Own Story ~

My food obsession began long before I knew the word "diet." I looked at my thighs when I was eight years old and saw the fat. I was horrified. I understood why friends made fun of me. Even adults made fun of me. On a picnic with other families, one of the fathers asked me if I would like some potato chips, as he gestured for me to take some. I answered, "No," somehow knowing at that young age that I should not be eating potato chips. But then came the laughter from an insensitive family friend as he shouted, "You don't look like you don't eat potato chips!" I heard everyone laughing. Recalling the incident still makes me cry.

Not only did I discover at the age of eight that I was fat, I discovered that I was not safe anymore. After all, adults were supposed to be kind, and a refuge from the insults of children. That thoughtless, heartless man set me straight and my innocent view of the world was shattered.

I became a closet eater, probably among the youngest in history. I became so aware that there were foods that I shouldn't eat that I assumed everyone was watching my plate. There were endless glances, smirks, and comments about my

3

weight. Even kids next to me at a party would make me feel self-conscious about eating birthday cake.

It's so sad that people didn't hesitate to call me chubby, so sad that they would say, "Should you be eating that?" Even my grandmother would come to visit with bags of homemade goodies of pastries and cookies, and bags of nuts and treats. And the comment was always the same, "Those are for your brothers." That is, not for me. Not for the child who couldn't afford to eat a cookie. Not for the child who got the "fat gene."

The result was only eating "diet food" in public. But the "adjusted eating habits" were also met with judgment. "Oh, you're being so good!" And I wasn't "good" when I was eating cake? And I was "good" when I ate carrots and celery sticks? I allowed people to destroy my self-view, and my perception of myself grew darker and darker. This was the 1960's when Twiggy, Lesley Hornby, five years older than me, was the rage. Overnight, she became the look of the minute. She was a skinny, rail-thin superstar. Models became taller and thinner while I became fatter and fatter. I began to interpret the attention for these skinny models as love. I began to think that love was reserved for skinny people.

The television, magazine, and billboard explosion only glorified and heightened the importance of these characteristics into my consciousness. Never before were women so tall, so slim, and so perfect. Images, images, and more images. Perfect people and perfect lives. They were the ones who belonged to love and love belonged to them. They were loved and they were lovable. Because they were skinny, right?

Even doctors exacerbated my low self-image. The pediatrician poked his finger in my belly during check-ups and laughed. At recess, I stood on line and didn't play with the other children for fear they would make fun of me. As I grew fatter, I grew quieter. I went through periods of isolation. In the seventh grade, because I had befriended a less popular girl in school, my name and weight was scribbled on the hallway walls. I was mortified. At my yearly physical, when I was sixteen years old, my doctor commented that I was the perfect weight; for a six-foot-two basketball player. As a pregnant woman, my doctor commented that I had gained too much weight that month. I told him that I was watching what I ate. He looked at me and said, "You're watching alright. You're watching everything go into your mouth."

You can't make up these stories. Sadly, they are all true.

In elementary school, during lunch period, nobody bothered with me. I ate all of my food. The skinny kids who didn't like to eat got all the attention. I witnessed the attention teachers heaped on them while trying to cajole them to take one bite or one sip. I was like a fly on the wall, just watching. I started to feel more and more comfortable in my own little world. I become more and more numb because the pain was too great. I was almost forty years old when I began to shed the layers of fat just to reveal the pain beneath.

I hated myself. I began to believe that I would never have a "normal" female figure. The emphasis on weight only made me long for a skinny body even more. The starvation followed. I was too young to know how to diet, what food choices to make, and what portion control was all about. I only knew from reading articles in magazines in the drugstore that lettuce seemed to be a diet food. I went days on end only eating lettuce. No wonder that I felt lightheaded and sick!

Then the "Monday morning syndrome" began. I have no idea where that came from but if I broke my diet on Tuesday, I would stuff my face until the next Monday when I would start another diet, promising myself to never, ever eat fattening food again. Many Monday mornings came and went through my life, not being able to stay in control and I just became fatter and fatter.

Through it all, I only wanted one thing; to be skinny. Skinny meant popularity. Skinny meant people loving you and admiring you. Skinny meant no comments or insults. I wanted to be skinny more than anything in the world. I wanted the willpower to get skinny. But I couldn't manage to stop eating. To me, the only way to become skinny was to starve myself and starving led to bingeing. Starving and bingeing lasted for many years.

By the time I was thirty-eight years old, my weight crept up to 233.5 pounds. I am five feet three inches tall. I wanted to die. I had everything a woman could want - a husband and children, a house without a mortgage, a backyard and a swing set, two cars, and a wonderful community. Yet, I hated myself. It was painful to walk into a room full of people. I felt, whether imagined or not, that everyone was thinking, "I can't believe how much weight Rivka gained! I can't believe she got so fat!" I couldn't believe it, either.

I tried to be a normal person. I was active in my community and had many friends. I tried to overcome my shame and pushed myself to attend synagogue services every Saturday morning. I took my kids to the local swim club and playground to be with other children, even though I did not want to be seen in public.

I felt that I was always the fattest person in the room. I probably was. I was miserable. And then three things happened.

Firstly, even though I obeyed all the laws of my religion, it never occurred to me that G-d was aware of me. I was aware of Him, but I felt so insignificant, how could G-d give me a moment's notice? Divine Providence intervened when I met a woman at an over-eater's meeting. She was older and single. She announced that she had taken off a tremendous amount of weight. I was waiting for the punch line when she said, "G-d loves me." I listened as she described her one-on-one connection to G-d and how He helped her lose weight. It never occurred to me that G-d loved me. It never occurred to me that I could talk directly to G-d. It never occurred to me that G-d could help me lose weight. My relationship with G-d changed at that moment.

Secondly, I got a call from one of my brothers who is an anesthesiologist and did many cardiac cases. He gently told me, "You know, I have women your age who have heart attacks on the operating table." All the while I was numbing myself with food, it never occurred to me that I was also destroying my health.

Thirdly, but certainly not the least, was that I found my best friend, my soul sister. We met at a charity function on a Sunday afternoon. The next morning and every single morning thereafter, she called me. To this day, I joke with her that she is the one giving 100% to the relationship. It was life changing. We could talk about anything and everything. And boy, did we! And we still do! She made me feel that she cared about me and that I was important. She reassures me that it's not a one-way street.

Chapter
~ 1 ~

"Write Your Own Story"

1. When did you start struggling with your weight?

2. Were you an overweight child or did you gain the weight later in life?

3. Describe how being overweight has affected your life.

4. What needs to happen in your life, to switch from complaining and feeling miserable about being overweight, to making losing weight the most important thing in your life?

5. Journal here how you believe you can start losing weight.

Chapter
~ 2 ~

Mistakes I Made Along the Way

~ What Kept Me in Yo-Yo Mode

for More than Forty years~

Food was my best friend. It was always there for me. It was always available. Life experiences shaped many of the circumstances I found myself in. These were not my choice, but how I reacted to them was. Whereas someone else could have been as lonely as I was, they would not have made the mistake of using food to soothe them. But I did. Only looking back do I see that I used food as a band-aid for anything and everything. I used food to fill the voids in my life. That was a huge mistake.

I used food to fill loneliness. As a child, I attended a private school out of the community. No one else in my town attended that school, so I had few local friends to play with. I only had brothers who didn't play with dolls. As a result, I spent most of my time alone in my room.

In college, I still lived at home and drove to a city college about ten miles away. Most of my college friends lived close to school and hung out in the cafeteria after classes. I had to go to work for spending money, so I didn't have that luxury.

After college, I went to work as a secretary. I lived alone in a studio apartment in Manhattan.

I was lonely. Really, really lonely.

Then, I met a guy, dated for ten months, got engaged and got married six weeks later. We moved into his apartment. I didn't know a soul.

Most of my friends had also gotten married, moved away and were busy with their own lives. In those days, the further the distance, the more the phone call would cost. Hard to imagine, right? But on our newlywed budget it was not possible to call out-of-state friends. I was lonely. I gained fifty pounds in my first year of marriage.

Two years later, we moved to New Jersey with our four month old daughter, to a community where I did not know anyone. We could not afford a second car so I was stuck at home with an infant. I was miserable for years and continued gaining weight.

I turned to food when I felt deprived. I first experienced this emotion when I was a child. I lived in a nice neighborhood that my parents could not afford. I was too young to understand that they moved here because they wanted the best for us. All I knew was that my clothing was bought two sizes too big so that they'd fit longer. I felt dumpy and even fatter with those ill-fitting clothes. I had very few toys. The children on the block seemed to have tons of toys. It was hard for me to stop feeling sorry for myself. Feeling deprived made me very unhappy. Feeling unhappy made me eat.

I ate when I could not express myself. I grew up in a time when "Children should be seen and not heard." I was never allowed to express my emotions and, therefore, never voiced an opinion. As a result, I became an emotional eater. Then I started to associate even positive emotions with eating.

It got to a point that even feeling excited about something good would trigger eating. I was eating all the time. All emotions led to food. If I "felt," I ate. I was on a path of self-destruction.

Being overweight ruined my self-esteem. On the one hand, I wanted to lose weight desperately, but on the other hand, I felt I did not deserve to be thin. This was compounded with the issue of perfectionism which would always creep in and set me up for failure. Unhealthy, unsustainable diets became the rage and I tried all of them. Of course, I would not be able to stick perfectly to a diet of cabbage soup and hard-boiled eggs. Who could for any period of time? But I expected perfection. I would fail and revert to the old habits of poor food choices and large portions. Once again, I beat myself up. Beating myself up made me feel miserable. I felt miserable. I ate.

I used to weigh and measure all of my food. I even brought a scale to restaurants adding to the stigma of being overweight. Common sense left me. I never asked what does my body need? I was just following rules that someone else decided. No voice! I had to learn to listen to myself and figure out which foods and portion sizes worked best for me.

I hated my body and wanted to be the exact opposite of my body-type. I was sure that if I was in another woman's body –

a tall, skinny body – then I'd be happy. I had to learn that beauty comes in many shapes and sizes. Wishing I looked different was self-defeating.

Weight loss success only came once I accepted myself just as I was. Actually, even more than that. I started losing weight when I began to appreciate the positive things about my figure. I also began to focus on being grateful that my body functioned normally. I had legs that could walk and dance, arms that could hold a baby, and breasts that could nurse a child. I matured and now love everything about my body – well, almost everything.

Chapter
~ 2 ~

"Write Your Own Story"

1. Do you have friends? If so, are you happy with those relationships?

2. Are you isolated?

3. Do you need friends? If so, how do you think you can make friends?

4. Do you go to the gym, attend any exercise classes, etc.?

5. Are you comfortable being alone?

6. Are you an emotional eater?

7. How can you be kinder to yourself?

8. Can you learn from your mistakes?

9. How can you develop healthy eating habits?

10. Can you accept and appreciate your body?

Chapter
~ 3 ~

What I Did to Lose Weight

~ Strategies that Worked ~

Creating my goals and defining their supporting steps were an integral part of my journey. Let me explain. I kept wishing I would lose weight. I kept thinking I wanted to lose weight. I kept complaining that I could not lose weight. I finally started to lose weight when I created a plan. Sounds like a lot of work? It was. It was worth it. So how do you start?

When you want to achieve anything in life, do you just sit back and wait for it to happen? Do you wish and think it would be great if such and such would occur or just drift right into my life? In any area you choose, would you succeed without any effort?

Here is an analogy to give a glimpse of how ridiculous it is to try to achieve anything without having a plan. A plan needs to be created with specific goals and steps to achieve those goals.

Imagine a businessman. He rents an office. He goes to the local office equipment store and buys out the store. From pens and pencils, computers and printers, he's got it all. Shiny new desks arrive. Swivel leather chairs. The phone company installed the latest and greatest most sophisticated phone system ever. The cable company set up Wi-Fi.

He hired top-notch employees. He even put a dress code into place. He went to the office every day and sat in his black leather chair. The businessman sat with the idea of a successful business, wishing he would make bazillions of dollars. He thinks everything is great. After awhile, he starts wondering why he hasn't made any money.

Any wonder? He forgot to create a business plan. He forgot to decide which specific business to go into. He completely glossed over defining his goals. Without knowing his goals, he could not create the steps to reach them. Sounds ridiculous, doesn't it?

But that is exactly what I did when I wanted to lose weight. It was nothing more than wishful thinking.

I had the desire to lose weight. I wished to lose weight. I wanted to lose weight. I ached to be slimmer.
I failed because I didn't define my goals explicitly. Saying I wanted to lose weight was too vague. To make this crystal clear, here are my personal, current goals and the steps to achieve them:

GOAL – Lower my blood pressure.
    Steps:
      1. Meditate 10 minutes every day.
      2. Avoid very salty foods.
      3. Exercise for a minimum of 30 minutes 5 days a week.

GOAL – Maintain current weight.

Steps:
1. Exercise for a minimum of 30 minutes 5 days a week.
2. Journal every morning.
3. Maintain my 90/10 eating rule. 90% eat healthy food, 10% eat whatever I want (in reasonable portions)
4. Keep up my friendships!

Here are more examples of general goals and steps.

GOAL – Wearing that snug dress for my dinner date next month.
   Steps:
   1. Cut my breakfast muffin in half.
   2. Exercise three days a week.

GOAL – Enjoy shopping for clothes.
   Steps:
   1. Not taking seconds of the starchy foods at meals.
   2. Limiting myself to one glass of wine with dinner.

GOAL – Eating out with friends and not being frantic over what I should/could eat.
   Steps:
   1. Call the restaurant ahead of time and decide what to eat before I go.
   2. Eat a salad before I go so I am not ravenous when I get to the restaurant.

GOAL – Weigh the same as my wedding day.
   Steps:
   1. Create a food plan.
   2. Eliminate sugar and white flour.
   3. Exercise four times a week, 2x aerobic, 2x weight

training.

4. Drink more water.

GOAL – Enjoy exercise.
Steps:
1. Look for free trial classes at local gyms.
2. Put on music at home and just dance!
3. Try different exercise routines on YouTube.

GOAL – Fit exercise into my schedule.
Steps:
1. Schedule an exercise "appointment" on my calendar.
2. Determine what time works best for me.
3. If I keep missing my "appointment," adjust the time.

GOAL – Eat sitting down.
Steps:
1. Paste notes on kitchen cabinets, "I will only eat sitting down."
2. Enlist help from others. Give them permission to remind me to sit down if they catch me eating standing up.

These examples of goals and steps help you realize how important it is to determine a specific goal and then create the supporting steps. Notice how the goal, "Weigh the same as my wedding day," is much more concrete than saying, "I want to lose weight."

These goals and steps enabled me to own my behavior and my choices, leading to success.

Here is why it worked so well and continues to work for me. While I was losing weight, my goal was to become a healthy weight. One of the steps was to cut out white sugar. When I was faced with a slice of birthday cake, it registered, "Eliminating sugar is on the list of steps to reach my goal of becoming a healthy weight." So I chose not to eat the cake. It released me from the struggle. It freed me from any further conversation in my head. Eliminating sugar was one of my steps. Not only was there no conversation, no struggle or "war" in my head; it didn't even begin!

See the difference? I was not in a "poor-me-I-can't-eat-the-cake" pity party. I behaved like an adult, taking charge of my life and my health. I made the wise decision to stick to the step that ultimately brought me satisfaction in the reward of reaching my healthy weight.

I did not say any of this is easy. I will say that it is all worth it.

Now I had to find the right support. That was kind of scary because it meant putting myself out there. Staying home and bemoaning my fat genes did not get me anywhere. Doing it alone, whether with a diet center, diet counselor or diet doctor – it was still just me, myself and I when I came home from my weekly visit, until my next weigh-in. Isolated. Just me and my food plan; no support for approximately 167 ½ hours per week (a week has 168 hours, so let's say my diet doctor appointment was at most half an hour).

I realized I needed support in-between my visits. I needed someone to turn to when my children's leftovers screamed, "Eat me," even from the garbage. I needed someone to turn to when I got upset. When I was still sitting on the sofa, I needed someone to turn to for encouragement to get up and keep my 2:00 pm exercise appointment.

Where could I find like-minded people? I asked around and found a group of women struggling with the same issues. I had my 167 ½ hours of isolation finally covered! There was support almost every hour of every day. We met once a week. We exchanged our phone numbers and what hours of the day we were available to receive calls. With this information, I never had to hesitate if I needed help in the middle of the night because I knew who was up! I went to my list. Knowing that at every turn I would have someone who would listen and someone to talk to for support, made a big difference. I was no longer alone.

Having support was so much deeper than just being able to call someone at 3:00 am. I also found people I could trust. These women mirrored my flaws, gently letting me know what I could not see for myself. They helped me with so much more than just healthy eating. They taught me to let go of situations that caused me stress, because being stressed always led me to overeat. Here are some examples. They made me realize I was being too nice for my own good. I was taught to be a good girl and always be "nice." I bring up this example here because had it not been for the support of these wonderful women it would not have occurred to me to I could drop a toxic relationship. That's exactly what I learned to do with their help, among many other things. I developed new friendships with like-minded people while edging out relationships that no longer served me. It was not easy, but something I needed to do for my own sanity. I had to get over the guilt. Their support kept me strong. I could never have gotten through it alone. I removed isolation by developing and enriching these new relationships. No one was more than a phone call away.

Enlarging my circle of friends brings me to my next topic - hanging out with happy people. You know the expression, "Misery loves company?" On some level, I believe I drew these people to me. I used to feel an obligation to be the one to remove them from their anguish until I realized that not only was I not helping them, I was hurting myself. Being with naysayers, people that were always negative and complaining dragged me into their world. I would listen to them gripe about everything. I didn't enjoy being with them and found I was even drawn into their unhealthy mindsets. Just being with them made me focus on what was wrong in my life. I had to stop that nonsense.

The absolute opposite is true, too. I found that happiness increases happiness. I paid attention to the people that smiled and laughed a lot. They were so much more fun to be with! I befriended couples with strong, healthy marriages. I associated with people who wanted to fill their lives with joy. Happiness and joy are like lighting a candle. When you light one candle from another, you increase the light. The light becomes brighter with every new candle you light. This is exactly how I felt when I began to spend time with happy people. Our cheerfulness played on each other, increasing smiles all around. I look for friends that are interesting, love to learn and grow, and know how to enjoy life. What a difference!

A new-found confidence was the outcome of all the changes I had made. I slowly began to have regard for my thoughts, feelings, and needs. I slowly began speaking up for myself.

There were some people that were quite disturbed with the new me. I was no longer a doormat. If something bothered me, I was able to find my voice and say what I had to say, saying it nicely. I learned that I am entitled to my opinion and at the same time, I allow you to have your opinion. We don't have to agree. I've learned to "agree to disagree." You can think what you want, behave the way you want, as long as I am not hurt in the process. I learned to come at situations with more of a posture of curiosity. Instead of thinking, "How could she possibly do, think or believe that!?" – now I question. "That's so interesting. Please tell me how you came to that decision?" Coming from a position of wanting to understand where someone else is coming from has given me freedom. It reduces anxiety in many situations. Instead of putting the other person on the defensive, I can own my opinion or way of doing things, inquire as to yours, and let us each operate the way that is best for ourselves, respecting each other's differences.

Sometimes, a situation is not even worth discussing, but better off discarding. For example, in the past, if someone said something that hurt me (intentionally or unintentionally), I would react, "I can't believe he/she said that? How could they treat me that way?" I would allow them to have an impact on me. Today I say to myself, "I may not like the words that person said to me, and their words may be hurtful, but I will not allow myself to be hurt." I am in control of my emotions. I choose not to allow it to bother me. I need to do this for myself.

The first way, the way I used to respond, was what drove me to eat to deal with the hurt. What I do now, is acknowledge the feelings and the words, and then let it go. The longer you practice this, the easier it becomes your default behavior. Just release those words and make your best attempt to say, "Who cares?" When you hold onto hurtful words, you are giving that other person power over you. They do not deserve it. Do not give it to them! If you can't "get over" it yourself, call an understanding friend for advice, comfort, and support. There are still those times, but thankfully few and far between, when someone will really use me as their target. If I can't handle it myself, I promptly pick up the phone and call a supportive friend for advice.

I changed what was possible to change, accepted with grace anything in my life I could not change and removed myself from those people and situations that were unacceptable. I decided to no longer hurt myself.

Now for the topic of food. It is almost too simple; I shudder at how long it took me just to "get it." Just eat! Now hold on, I didn't say gorge and I didn't say binge. I said, "Just eat." I began to notice that slim friends never made conscious food choices. They didn't even know how many calories were in an orange! How could that be? If they didn't know how many calories a food had, how could they possibly know how much to eat, which food to eat, when to eat? I paid thousands of dollars through the years to have people tell me which foods I was allowed to eat, how to prepare them, when to eat and how much of each food to eat.

Insanity? You bet. The food plans, the measuring cups, the measuring spoons, the scales, the calorie-count books, the rules, of every plan I followed, are a thing of the past. They never worked for the long term.

Here's the secret. Here is how those naturally slim friends never had to know how many calories were in each food or how much of a food to eat. They listen to themselves. They pay attention if they are full. They don't need to measure half-a-cup of this or half-a-cup of that. When losing weight became easier for me, it was because I started paying attention. Period. I slowed down when I ate. I chewed my food when I ate. I noticed when I was full. I gave myself time to eat instead of shoveling it in. If I did not have at least fifteen minutes to eat a meal, I chose not to eat. I waited until I could enjoy my food, giving myself a chance to notice when I felt satisfied.

Slim people decide what to eat based on what they are in the mood for. They don't have to stuff in any particular fattening food because they may never have the chance again to eat it. They don't categorize food into prohibited and non-prohibited. They just eat. They listen to themselves.

I learned to listen to myself, too. I am not a small eater and teeny-tiny portions never satisfied my appetite. I started using common sense. If I needed larger portions and I wanted to lose weight, what did I need to do? Bingo. You guessed it. I ate my larger portions of food from the vegetable and salad categories. Sometimes I am embarrassed when eating with friends or family because I eat really large salads. But what makes them so large? The greens. The lettuces. I fill most of my plate with a bed of lettuces; arugula, baby romaine, spinach, parsley, etc. Then come the chopped cucumbers, raw colorful peppers, etc. Next comes adding the highest calorie foods, like the protein, in a modest portion. Then I give a quick pour of healthy oil and lots of spices. Sandwiches appear embarrassingly huge because of the amount of salad in them. On top of my protein, I stack, and I mean stack, thinly sliced layers of cucumbers, tomatoes, raw zucchini and herbs. If I opt for a nut butter and jelly sandwich, I always make certain to enjoy it with a salad or a bowl of soup. A simple sandwich would not be enough.

But I was careful. Here is a critical point. I never allowed myself to feel stuffed. Part of my success was learning to get away from needing to feel so full every time I walked away from the table.

These changes did not happen overnight. I was determined to listen to myself. I had to have patience until I began to intuitively know what to eat. I had to determine what portion sizes worked for me and not for someone else. I learned how to measure in my mind and understand that some days I needed more food and some days I needed less. It is not an exact science. I failed miserably every time someone else told me how much to eat. Why? There are two reasons. Firstly, if I didn't follow the plan perfectly I berated myself and got depressed. If I was told to eat half-a-cup of brown rice, but wasn't satisfied and took another carefully measured portion, I got upset because I "went off" my diet. That just led to more overeating! Secondly, half-a-cup of anything never did it for me. A one-cup portion at one meal per day better filled my personal needs. Till today, I will sooner eat an entire sandwich, two slices of bread at a meal, rather than one slice at two meals. If you are reading this book, I would venture to say that measuring has not worked for you, either.

I actually experienced being handed a sheet of paper that said, "One-cup of lettuce, a quarter-of-a-cup of yellow peppers (I was told that red peppers had too much starch in them), one small cucumber and two thin slices of tomato." I laugh when I look back and remember that I actually did this over and over and over again. Thin slices of tomato! I measured iceberg lettuce in measuring cups. I actually paid for people to tell me to eat one-sixth of an avocado because more "has too many calories." A red flag should have gone up when those same diet counselors allowed me to eat "100-calorie packs" of completely nutrient-deficient snack bags. Was there something wrong with this picture? There certainly was. I was so busy listening to what others told me I should be eating when I should have been figuring it out for myself. My needs are not the same as yours. Yours are not the same as mine. Experiment and see for yourself what works for you and what does not.

Of course, I had to be savvy and smart when it came to high-calorie foods. I divided them into healthy and not-so-healthy categories. If it was real food, like an avocado, I sliced it open and ate an entire half. When it came to pizza or bagels, I tried to reduce the number of times a week I ate those foods, and when I did choose to eat them, I ate half the amount I used to eat.

A really interesting thing happened when I started to do this. The more I ate those foods, by allowing myself to eat them, the fainter the desire to eat them became. It became so simple. This goes all the way back to the Garden of Eden adage "forbidden fruit." When I never allowed myself a particular food, you guessed it, that would be the one I would dream about and salivate over. I started allowing myself to eat almost everything. I did cut out the sugar and white flour so when I say bagel, I cut out white flour bagels. I ate a whole wheat or pumpernickel one.

In the past I thought I could not possibly give up pizza. I could not understand how anyone could resist eating pizza while doling it out to their kids or sitting in a pizza shop with them, sipping a bottle of water and not eating any. By telling myself that I can have pizza whenever I want, again, my desire diminished. When I do eat it, I have a slice, one slice, because I can have it again! I also make the best possible choice when it comes to pizza. My best choice is a thin, whole-wheat crust pizza, light on the cheese. I add vegetables on top, too.

I try to prepare the same foods in healthier ways. Eggplant parmesan is made with slices of baked eggplant, lots of additional vegetables, no-sugar added tomato sauce, and very little cheese. Fried chicken is dipped lightly in oil, dredged through some crushed healthy cereal and baked in the oven. After so many years of being told to eat bland foods that I did not even enjoy, making my food delicious is of utmost importance. I found that the tastier my food was, the more I enjoyed it. The more I enjoyed it, the faster I became satisfied and therefore, the less I needed to eat.

In my private coaching practice, I find that knowing what to snack on is a big challenge. Our ideas of snacking have been corrupted from advertising and commercials. When clients ask me what I snack on I tell them, "Oranges, kiwis, nuts, smoothies, green tea, figs, pepper strips, baby carrots. Lots of things!"

I can pretty much say that almost 100% of the time, I get the same reply. "No, but what do you *snack* on?"

Television commercials and print ads for unhealthy foods are destroying our health. Our nation has unprecedented obesity, cancer, heart attack and diabetes rates. Doesn't it sadden you to know that Adult Onset Diabetes has been renamed to Diabetes II, because children at younger and younger ages have been diagnosed with diabetes? We are a society that is bombarded with messages that snacks are potato chips, pretzels, and frozen boxes that are popped into a microwave. These same foods are the ones that are creating the frightening rise of medical issues.

I changed my mindset when it came to snacking. I tried to go from meal to meal, but if I was hungry, I ate. I didn't plan to snack once, twice or three times a day. When clients ask me how many snacks a day they can have, my answer is always the same. "I don't know." They look at me quizzically, and ask, "Aren't you my Health Coach, lady?" Exactly, I am your Health Coach. I am trying to teach you to notice if you need a snack, or is it really some other need you are trying to fill at that moment. I am coaxing you with questions as to whether you truly need to eat. So to answer the question of snacking, I snack if I'm very hungry and it's still more than an hour till the next meal. What do I snack on? Whatever I'm in the mood for. I try to balance my nutrition, thinking about my whole day's food. If I am having a higher calorie meal for dinner, I naturally take a lower calorie snack. If I am having a lighter dinner, I might eat a bar made from nuts and dates, a higher calorie snack. Choose bars that are made only from ingredients like dates, nuts and fruit. Or I may snack on a handful of nuts, a fruit or raw vegetables. I also ask myself, "What will nourish me?" Isn't that what food is for? Keeping this in the forefront of my mind empowers me to make smart choices. I also find that a mini-meal can be very satisfying. I enjoy half a portion of a favorite breakfast or lunch. Sometimes I save some of my morning smoothie. It's not what I eat each meal and each snack. I try to look at the whole picture. I take into account the day before and the next day, not only the food for that day.

I also wanted to make sure that I ate enough. Sound crazy? Here I am sharing what I did to lose weight and then I tell you not to slash calories. Exactly. When I cut my calories back too much, my body went into preservation mode. It slowed my metabolism, so I needed even fewer calories to maintain the same weight! We humans are built that way. It's called survival. So eating enough is important. I did not want to get my body used to so few calories that I would have to live off of celery sticks and skimmed-milk cottage cheese the rest of my life.

Eating in restaurants was a big challenge. I was a housewife. I planned, shopped, cooked and cleaned up from every single meal. It was nice to have a break once in awhile. But I lost control and over-ate every single time I went to a restaurant. I easily fell into the trap of ordering the wrong foods and devouring the entire bread basket. I didn't want to give up going out to eat. I told myself that if I got out of control in restaurants I would not treat myself to this pleasure in life. I had to develop a plan.

My new approach worked like a charm. In the past, I perused the menu. I salivated just reading it. This set me up for failure because baked ziti with fries was too great a temptation. This had to change, so instead of deciding what to eat when I got to the restaurant, I called ahead and planned before I arrived. This was before computers. Now I go to the restaurant's website to make my choice and I stick to it when I get there. I overcame the first obstacle. The next challenge was sticking to my decision. If someone at my table ordered something fattening, I was tempted to order the same. So I always ordered first and did not allow myself to change my order. This also reinforced eating what I was in the mood food, rather than being swayed by someone else's choice. I overcame the second obstacle.

In addition to these two strategies, upon being seated, I handed the bread basket to the waiter. I saved myself hundreds of calories. These three changes alone made eating out a real treat. I got a break from the kitchen. I spent quality time with family and friends. Most of all, I left the restaurant feeling good about myself.

Now here is how I figured out how to maintain my weight while vacationing. If I went away for a few days, a week or a month, the strategy was always the same. I did my research before I left. I made sure fruit and salad were available; I researched where I could buy them and made sure I rented a refrigerator for my room. I ate lots of salad and vegetables with protein. For snacks, I brought single portions of whole-grain crackers, nuts or some of my favorite bars in mini-sized portions. They were always in my purse.

Another strategy for success on vacation is that I allowed myself to eat whatever I wanted at the last meal, including dessert. I tried doing the same exact thing, other than the timing and always failed. If I had this meal and dessert any other day, I had trouble getting back on track. Why does this work? When I had this meal and dessert at the last meal of vacation, I easily got back on track when I got home because

32

I changed my environment. I went straight back to my normal routine. It worked like a charm, every single time and it still does.

Now with food choices in place, I had to start moving. I had to start exercising. It was not easy because of my weight. I could not do much at first because the stress was too great on my knees and joints. What kept me motivated was keeping in mind that I was improving my health along with my physical appearance.

Exercise did not necessarily mean formal. I did not join a gym at first. I was too embarrassed. It did not mean spending a fortune on exercise equipment or pumping weights for hours.
It did mean finding ways of moving more and sitting less! I started slowly. When I did too much, too soon, it only backfired. When I over-exercised, I got so sore that it was days until I could exercise again. I started walking for just a few blocks and built up the distance. After a few months, I was walking miles at a time, looking forward to waking up in the morning in anticipation of my daily walk. Instead of parking close to my destinations, I parked a few blocks away. I heard this advice many times before, but now I actually did it. The domino effect occurred. Moving more propelled further physical activity. Instead of taking an elevator, I got off one or two floors before the floor I needed and walked up those few flights of stairs. You get the picture. I just started moving!

I once read a study with two Control Groups. Group A was told to exercise 30 minutes a day and Group B was told to exercise ten minutes, three times a day. Can you guess which group had the most accumulated minutes of exercising over the course of the week? Group B added up more time than Group A because too often people in Group A could not find an entire 30 minutes to devote to exercise. Group B easily found ten minutes if not once, but even two or three times a day, adding up to more cumulative minutes than Group A. They had more success in improving their health! In the past, when I struggled to lose weight, I wouldn't exercise at all if I didn't have an hour.

I took this to heart. On days I didn't fit in exercise, I made it my business to go up and down the staircase in my house a few extra times, going up fast! Now I will walk or dance around the house for only ten minutes. Those ten minutes really add up. A funny thing frequently occurred when I forced myself to walk for ten minutes. I inevitably walked longer. I usually enjoyed myself so much that I spent much longer ten minutes. Music was also great in getting me off my derriere. Often, when I thought I was too tired to exercise, I put on some music and "Hey, where did all that energy come from? A moment ago I couldn't think of putting one foot in front of the other, even to go to the refrigerator!" Then I was dancing!

I also used to think that I could never exercise at night. I started exercising at night and it was great. For years, I tried to exercise during the day. During the day, so many things had to be taken care of. In the evening, things would wind down and I was able to commit to exercising. In fact, the days I exercised in the evenings, I ate less at dinner, knowing that I could not exercise on a full stomach.

I was losing weight, I was feeling great and I was exercising. I plateaued after losing fifty pounds. Depression was not the word for what I experienced. I needed to lose another fifty pounds! What happened? Wasn't I doing great? The weight came off slowly and then to a complete standstill. I could not figure out what was going on. I exercised more. The scale did not budge. This went on for months. I stuck to my healthy eating. I increased the time and number of days doing aerobics.

A few more months went by. I was stuck between a rock and a hard place. I could not blame external factors on the sudden halt in my weight loss. There were no out of the ordinary stresses in my life. No changes in my eating or exercising. What was going on? The situation was difficult. If I gave up, slacking off my food and exercise routine, I would only gain weight. If I cut my calories back, I would slow down my metabolism. I already increased my exercise to seven days a week. I went for blood work. Something had to be wrong. The blood work came back normal. Normal? What's normal about being more than fifty pounds overweight, exercising for an hour a day and eating properly? The scale didn't budge.

Then I read an article in a magazine. I knew very little about weight training. I thought it was solely for men and if a woman lifted weights, she would bulk up. I knew nothing! When I learned that a pound of muscle burns more fat at rest than a pound of fat at rest, I ran, not walked, to my local gym. I hired a trainer immediately. In order to improve my metabolism, I worked extra hard. I started weight training three days a week. In addition to the weight training, I continued my walks at least four to five days a week. For months, I did not miss a day. Not only was I physically exercising, I experienced an exercise in patience.

One month later, no change on the scale. My trainer gave me much-needed encouragement. Two months later I got on the scale. I weighed the same. I was ready to give up. Again, my trainer cheered me on and begged me to stay on track because he said I looked leaner. After about three months, when I really started to get frustrated, the scale started moving. I was so excited. Weight training was critical in firing up my metabolism. The reward for my tremendous efforts was finally paying off. I was thrilled to see the scale moving downwards again. The weight loss was slow and steady until I finally reached my goal.

Chapter
~ 3 ~

"Write Your Own Story"

1. Write down your goals and your steps.

2. Create your personal eating plan. What will help you listen to your body as to which foods you should be eating? How much? How often?

3. How will you find the right support?

4. How will you nurture the friendships that serve you best and remove the ones that don't?

5. How can you make peace with the unchangeable in your life and remove yourself from the unacceptable?

6. Which tips are you willing to try when dining out?

7. Will allowing yourself anything you want at the last meal on vacation work for you?

8. Are you exercising? Are you doing a variety of exercises?

Chapter
~ 4 ~

Audio Messages

~ Positive Thoughts & the Art of Relaxation ~

My unflattering self-image flooded my brain with pessimistic thoughts, setting me up for failure. I needed to believe that I was a worthy, important and lovable person in order to find success. I did not get that message from others. I had to learn those new messages by myself.

I was also high-strung and anxious, as a result of the frustration from repeated failures to lose weight.
How did I start flooding my brain with positive messages, with messages of love and acceptance? How did I reinforce being good to myself, when I never could in the past? How did I start to calm down?

Let me share my experience with the first doctor that actually began the process of rewiring my negative thoughts to positive, supportive ones, and how he taught me relaxation techniques.

When I was overweight, I scanned the cover of every single magazine for a diet promising successful weight loss. I checked the newest books to find the latest and greatest diet. Whenever a new diet doctor or diet center was mentioned, I excitedly hoped that it would be local enough for me to go to but I was inevitably disappointed because I lived in the New Jersey suburbs. Not exactly a place for a thriving weight-loss center.

But then one day I read an article about Dr. Fleischer, in the newest issue of a popular magazine. The article mentioned his amazing success with weight loss. Moreover, he was located in a town just a five-minute drive from home. I was ecstatic! I called and he fit me in that same night, on the weekend, on a Sunday night!

Dr. Nathan Fleischer was a very old man when I went to him. I still have the audio tape he made for me. The tape is dated May 19, 1985, making it more than thirty years ago. It was something I had never experienced before.

He was the first doctor to use audio messages, incorporating positive suggestions, complimenting me, mapping out a food plan, but most of all, allowing me to hear support any time of day or night. I could just pop the tape in my tape recorder, which I did, over and over again.

His words were soothing and calming, bringing me to a state of total relaxation. They gave me a newfound confidence that I could succeed.

Here is a transcription of the tape he made for me. Imagine it being spoken in a very tranquil and loving voice because that was the tone he used. In fact, till this day, when I play it, I feel like crying when he says my name. He said it with warmth, love and concern. He called me, "My dear." I was so starved for affection in my life, that even a stranger, a doctor that, of course, had no true feelings for me, could make me feel loved and cared for simply by saying my name.

Here are excerpts from the tape:

> Rivka, try making yourself as comfortable as you can right now and let me hear that deep sigh of relief. With your eyes closed, begin by relaxing your legs and let them go limp. Relax your arms and let them go limp just like two pieces of rope. Relax the muscles of the jaw so your teeth do not even touch. Feel that nice, easy feeling as your jaw relaxes and your arms relax and your legs relax. And now Rivka, relax the muscles around your eyes and when the muscles around your eyes are really relaxed, it will just seem as if you cannot open them.

> Relax the muscles around your eyes. And now, because the muscles around your eyes are so relaxed, it just seems as if you cannot open them. You can raise your eyebrows. It just seems as if you cannot open your eyes, so stop trying my dear. And now relax deeper and deeper and deeper. Breathe slowly and breathe deeply. With every easy breath you take, feel yourself relaxing deeper and deeper. It feels so good to relax. And now Rivka, while you are relaxing, I want you to imagine that you have made it. You look like a Junior Miss model.

> You feel wonderful, you look in the mirror and you're proud of yourself. And I say to you, Rivka, how do you feel now?

And you say, The impossible has occurred, Dr. Fleischer. I feel like a ballerina and I know I'll be this way as long as I live.

I say, What do you think really did it for you?

And you say, I simply followed your instructions. I changed my way of life completely. Now I don't have to hurt myself anymore. I feel wonderful being good to myself. I am following your food plan.

And now here is your meal plan. Yes, you get up in the morning and have either four ounces of tomato juice, a quarter of a cantaloupe or a two inch cut of any other melon. Your real treat is bran cereal. This is the only starch you will ever touch. You will carefully measure half a cup and add half a cup of non-fat milk. You can then have half a cup of skimmed-milk cottage cheese, eight ounces of plain yogurt, an egg, or one ounce of any other low-fat cheese. If you do not want the dairy or egg, you can have a piece of gefilte fish. If you don't want that, you can have three pieces of herring in wine sauce, or three and a half ounces of water-packed tuna, twice a week only. You can have all the coffee, all the tea, all the low-calorie drinks that you want. Lunch and dinner are the same. You can have four ounces of broiled, baked or roasted chicken or turkey. If you don't want that you can have four ounces of veal liver, beef liver, or chicken liver. Once in a great while you can even have filet mignon, roast beef or rib steak. Or have 6 ounces of either fillet of flounder, fillet of cod, fillet of rainbow trout or red snapper. And if you don't want that, you can always go back to your breakfast proteins, but you can have two pieces of gefilte fish, two eggs or six pieces of herring; the other protein portions are the same as breakfast. But you do know that a piece of roast beef or any other kind of beef is minimally 440 calories for 4 ounces, and 4 ounces of gefilte fish, maximally, 58 calories, and brook trout is maximally 65 calories. Take your choice. You also have your health salad. In addition to your lettuce, you can have chives, radishes, scallions, onions and even small slices of tomato. A piece of fruit is enjoyed after lunch or dinner. You can have either half a grapefruit, an orange, a tangerine, or better still a quarter of a cantaloupe, or a two-inch cut of any kind of melon. Isn't that beautiful?

For your snack, you must wait until anywhere between 3:00 and 4:30 in the afternoon. The snack is the same as your fruit after lunch and dinner. After dinner, if you wish, instead of having a fruit for dessert, you can have either an ice freeze or some sugar-free gelatin. Now if you want an ice freeze for dessert, you blend at least eight ice cubes, a 1/4 cup of water, a heaping teaspoon of skimmed-milk powder, a bag of artificial sweetener, and tablespoon of no-calorie flavoring. You have a delicious ice freeze. It's an imitation ice cream. And if you don't want that, you can have a popsicle. Fill your ice cube trays with diet soda, and while it's freezing, put toothpicks in the middle of every cube and have delicious popsicles that way. In-between meals, you can have all the bouillon, chicken, beef, vegetable or onion broth, that you want. Additionally, you can have all the celery, all the cucumber, all the hearts of lettuce you want. And you feel wonderful.

42

Now let's review the relaxation technique, a gentle lesson in the art of self-relaxation. Before every meal now, for as long as you live, you will take a minute or two and relax yourself.
Let's do it now together.

Rivka, take a deep breath in. And now my dear, with your eyes closed, you begin by relaxing your legs and you just let them go limp. You go up higher and relax your arms and relax the muscles of the jaw so that your teeth don't even touch. And now you relax the eye muscles so that you can raise your eyebrows, but your eyes do not open. You breathe slowly and easily as you say to yourself - I'm sensible. I'm sensible. I'm sensible.

When you say I am sensible, you think of a pleasant thought you will never forget. Think of a pleasant thought, dear. A beautiful thought. This will motivate you and make you happy. Think of your happiest moment in your life while saying I'm sensible. I'm sensible. I'm sensible. You're thinking of a happy, happy thought. And at this moment, you make up your mind precisely what you shall eat at this meal. Then you ask yourself why are you sensible.

You see a big, red neon sign on top of a mountain, that reads: Because. Because sugar and starch and fat and over-eating a gram more than I should eat are deadly, disgusting, nauseating poisons. So I don't begin. That's it. I don't begin. That's poison. Instead of the poison, I can have a popsicle (the frozen diet soda), I can have diet gelatin, bouillon, and broth. I can have celery, cucumber, hearts of lettuce, but I don't touch poison. I've got it made. And if ever I'm going to touch poison, I shall call my Dr. Fleischer no matter where he is in the world. I must talk to him before I put poison into my mouth. But I won't have to. Why? Because today I shall be perfect. I'm doing this for one day. Today I shall be perfect and then I don't begin. I don't begin and then I don't have any problem at all.

See yourself smiling. You're slender. You're graceful. You're smiling. You are beautiful and your therapist is so proud of you. I am truly proud of you, my dear. You are going to be slender as long as you live.
So now just very slowly count to yourself from one to three and when you reach three, my dear, you'll be wide awake, feeling so satisfied.

Tell yourself that you have everything in the world to live for and that you will be healthier with every passing day. Repeat over and over that you never felt better because you are taking off useless fat. Look in the mirror and say you are proud of yourself.
Now slowly count one, two, three and I open your eyes, feeling better than you have in a long time.

On side two of the tape, Dr. Fleischer starts with a comforting tone of voice but gets more demanding, as you will see by his words:

Alright Rivka, make yourself just as comfortable as you can right now and let me hear that deep sigh of relief. That's it.

And now, my dear, with your eyes closed, begin by relaxing your legs and let them go limp. And now, my dear, relax your arms, and let them go limp just like two pieces of rope. Relax the jaw muscles so that your teeth do not even touch. Feel that nice, easy feeling as the jaw relaxes and your arms relax, and your legs relax. Now, my dear, relax the muscles around your eyes and when the muscles around your eyes are really relaxed, it will just seem as if you cannot open them. Relax the muscles around your eyes and now because the muscles around your eyes are so relaxed, it just seems as if you cannot open them. You can raise your eyebrows, it just seems as if you cannot open your eyes so stop trying my dear, and now relax deeper and deeper and deeper. Breathe slowly and breathe deeply and with every deep, easy breath you take feel yourself relaxing deeper, and deeper. It feels so good to relax. And now, my dear, while you are relaxing, I want you to imagine that time has gone by and during this time, you've really learned to be good to yourself; you've learned to stop hurting yourself, you've learned to stop punishing yourself. You've really learned to eat sensibly.

Now you are returning to my office and as soon as you open that door I greet you. Rivka, it is so good to see you again! You look absolutely beautiful. Would you mind getting on that scale for me right now? And you say, Mind? It will be a pleasure and a joy Dr. Fleischer to get on that scale for you again. Don't you remember the first time I came to your office? Never

45

again in my life will I weigh that much. I hate to think about it.

I'll follow your program to the letter, the same as so many other thousands of others have done before me. I will reach a sensible weight goal. I've done just that. Here I am. What is my weight right now?
My dear, this is beautiful. What a strange coincidence. You have lost to the ounce, to the pound exactly as you wished!

Shall I put you on maintenance? And you say, Why should I go on maintenance, Dr. Fleischer? I'm still losing weight. When I stop losing weight, you'll put me on maintenance.

Rivka, my dear, you are just as intelligent as you are lovely and I'll do it your way. Whenever you want maintenance, just give me a phone call and I'll make a special appointment for you as we did on that Sunday evening when we started.
And you say, Doctor, it's almost too good to be true. Rivka dear, you learned, of course, that anything with sugar in it is poison. Candy, cookies, cake, pie, pastries, pudding, chocolate, ice cream, sherbet, custard, muffins, donuts.
They are all deadly, deadly poison. And just as deadly are the starches. Bread, rolls, crackers, bagels, potatoes, corn, all of the pastas, spaghetti, macaroni, pizza, ravioli, lasagna, ziti, potato chips and pretzels. Yes, all that junk is deadly poison. Anything with fats, salami, pastrami, corned beef, hamburgers, oil, margarine, mayonnaise and salad dressing. Any kind

of nuts, especially peanuts, peanut butter, cream cheese, jelly, jam. Any kind of cheese at all, except skimmed-milk cottage cheese, garden salad cottage cheese, or any 1% fat cheese is okay, but the others are deadly. Overeating is the worst poison of all. They'll take you to a hospital, they'll make you vomit, they'll make you wretch.

What comes up? All the sugars. All the starches. All the fats. Taste that vomit. Up your nose. All over your clothes. The worst vomit is overeating. Everything you overeat is vomit. It becomes vomit. They put a stomach pump on you. It's disgusting. You know you won't begin even if someone gives you a hundred million dollars to eat that way again. Your life is worth more. Your beauty is worth more. You don't begin. Instead of being a clumsy food addict, a fat addict, you have become graceful and slender and you enjoy it.

Dr. Fleischer was the forerunner, the beginning of my working on my mental state. He did something for me that was never accomplished. He taught me to flood myself with compliments. He made me believe that I could be slender. He made me believe I could reach my goal. He made me feel that as much as he would look successful if another client lost weight, he celebrated right alongside me, relishing my success as if I was his own daughter. He made me feel that he truly cared about me. No one else had ever done that before. He also used scare tactics. He called all those foods I shouldn't eat by their real name, "poison."

47

However, this was a long time ago and he didn't differentiate between healthy carbohydrates because that was the style of diets back then. I don't even think you could have found millet, brown rice or quinoa, at least not in any mainstream supermarkets in the mid-1980's. So he lumped all carbs and all oils together, even though now we can have these in moderation, in a healthy way. He did manage to shake me up a bit, by bringing to mind that overeating was deadly and that overeating would bring you to vomit. Not a pretty picture. Not the way I wanted to see myself.

He also was starting to make me aware of what was so obvious. He told me to stop hurting myself. I never viewed my overeating as psychologically harmful. I never realized that the way I abused myself with food reflected what I thought about myself. None of this was on a conscious level. I never got past, "I'm fat, I eat too much, I need to eat less and then I'll lose weight."

Another new thing that Dr. Fleischer taught me was to become aware before I ate. He was the first to tell me to breath and relax before a meal. He taught me to say, "Be sensible. Be sensible." Relaxation techniques were a new phenomenon, one that I was not familiar with. I never associated being anxious with over-eating. I never knew that in order to pay attention to and enjoy my food, I had to be in a calm, relaxed state.

He also taught me the value of support. Remember when he said to call him if I was ever having trouble? He gave me a new tool to break the vicious chain of getting upset and going straight to the food. Instead of going to the food, he taught me to pick up the phone and get help immediately, among the many other valuable lessons I learned from him.

Chapter
~ 4 ~

"Write Your Own Story"

1. What did you learn from Dr. Fleischer's tape?

2. What did you think about the food plan he gave me?

3. Do you give yourself positive messages?

4. Do you believe you can become slender and happy?

5. Do you have any relaxation techniques in place now?

Chapter
~ 5 ~

Cognitive Changes for Success

~ The Mind is a Powerful Aid ~

I was unaware I was trying to feed a hungry soul, not a hungry body. I was trying to self-medicate with food, which was not the cure for my ailments. It took me a long time to figure out that food masked my issues; it was my drug of choice to block out feelings. It was great at diverting attention away from difficult situations.

Focusing on food, eating food and then feeling guilty about eating food, left no time for me to say, "Hey, some things in my life are not so good. Let's deal with them," or "What do I need to change?" I was stuffing myself with donuts and bagels instead of asking for attention or hugs. Ever hear the expression "comfort food?" This is probably the greatest misnomer ever. Comfort? That was the last thing I got from stuffing my face. I experienced angst, self–loathing, and misery.

When I was lonely, I ate. When I was feeling abandoned or scared, I ate. When I felt criticized, I ate. When I was bored, I ate. When I felt unloved, I ate.

I ate a lot and I ate often. I turned to food for solace. It never delivered. I remember eating till I was so uncomfortably full that my stomach hurt. Why in the world did I eat that much? These poor eating habits were in full force at a very young age, way before I consciously associated unhappiness with eating. It didn't help that my father overate and was heavy, and my two brothers and mother could eat all they wanted and not gain a pound. I needed to eat less than anyone else in my family, and had no role models to give me a hint as to what was appropriate for a young girl.

I was acutely aware of the fattening food in the house. "Out of sight, out of mind," never worked for me. Those foods were always on my mind, even when stored in closed cupboards. I was drawn to those foods, like metal to a magnet. I knew they were there. I was aware of their presence. They took on a life of their own, not allowing me to choose otherwise. I could almost hear them speaking, "Eat me. I will make you feel better." Truly, I heard these foods talking to me. Their pull was so overwhelmingly strong, that I was a wimp without any hope in overcoming my addiction to them. It shut out the other voice, the one begging for help, the one asking me to get a grip and start working on my life. In comparison, this voice was a whisper.

The mind, body and spirit are not separate entities. What impacts one, impacts them all. I had to figure out the connection between how I perceived myself and how it played out in my life. It was futile to try to lose weight when my life was a mess. It's no wonder I was never successful in cutting back on my food when I was left unsatisfied in other areas. I put the cart before the horse. I dieted and dieted and then dieted some more. It didn't work. I could never sustain calorie restriction or exercise while my problems remained unsolved.

In retrospect, the reasons were pitiful. I blocked the truths of my life. I didn't allow myself to recognize my problems. It would have been too painful.

I had to develop new thought patterns to help reinforce my new healthy behaviors. I did this by focusing on the changes I needed to make in my life. I had a lot of work to do. I had a lot to learn.

Creating positive thoughts was vital in recovering from my food addiction, enabling me to create my best life ever! Changing my thoughts incorporated a one-hundred-and-eighty-degree turn away from non-productive, self-defeating beliefs. It was a win-win.

So what were my mind changes? I am now going to share many attitudes and beliefs that I turned around to serve me in a positive way. The shift in my thought processes brought everything I experienced to a positive light.

Learning how to function from a space of positivity and happiness was not natural for me. At times, the mental change felt more draining than an intense physical workout. I persevered. I worked on myself and then worked on myself some more because it dawned on me that if my mind was responsible for all the poor choices, maybe, just maybe, I can change things around by using it for better choices. My mind, which had initially been my enemy, ganging up against me with food on its' team, became my friend and powerful ally in staying away from what Dr. Fleischer taught me to call poison.

I used shifts in thinking to eventually get rid of my food addiction and explain why changing my thoughts were of utmost importance. Practicing them is like practicing anything else. Practice makes perfect and more automatic.

I started ditching the pity party and started operating with a new positive mindset. I rightfully blamed particular people in my life for not being there for me. I truly had unhappy experiences that would have driven a drunk to drink. I indulged in attending my own pity-party, dragging myself down in the process.

It also did not help that I was often accused of being too sensitive and overly emotional. Maybe I am sensitive and emotional. I learned that these also have many positive components. But, those words were *not* used with the intention of paying me a compliment. Accusations of, "Why are you getting so upset?" "Why can't you just let it roll off your back?" and "You're just like an elephant, you never forget!" swirled through my head. I was tormented by those words.

I consumed their words and believed I was not worth much at all. I gave credence to the wrong people and the wrong words. I let the ones that made fun of me flood my head with thoughts that I was not good enough. I allowed the comments of others to override objective self-assessment.

Living in that world of being hurt by others only made me miserable. All this negativity put my body into stress mode.

The adrenals release cortisol in this mode. The body is unable to distinguish between physical attack and mental attack. So when upset, the cortisol starts pumping. With all this cortisol being released, the metabolism simply cannot work efficiently; maybe that's another reason I could not lose weight. I was too often in stress-mode diminishing my body's ability to optimally burn calories.

By replacing old, self-defeating thoughts with positive ones, I ditched being a victim to being the luckiest girl in the world. I became peaceful, embracing my new-found positive perspective. Things were exactly the same – I just chose to view the same circumstances through a new lens. This was a major shift in my thinking. I began to view my unhappy childhood as the vehicle that created the strong woman that I am today. Had I been brought up with a silver spoon in my mouth, I never would have accomplished so much in my life. Those same experiences that were painful at the time shaped me into the person I am today. Pressure can produce fabulous results. Think of a diamond. Originally it was a piece of charcoal. Tremendous stress brings out its beauty.

The same thing occurred when I first starting eating healthier. I felt like I was being punished. This was another ploy of my "fat genes" trying to keep me fat. I felt really sorry for myself.

"Everyone else gets to eat yummy food and I have to eat plain salad and dry, broiled chicken. Why can't I go to take out places and eat those sandwiches with melted cheese oozing down the sides?" "Pizza, I can't live without pizza." "It's not fair!" I would complain to myself. "Why am I so unlucky?" I would lament silently to myself while sitting in a pizza shop, while sipping my diet soda. I would notice every single skinny person eating pizza, going deeper into my depression. Focusing on my deprivation set me into yet another binge when I got home, eating many more calories and doing way more damage than had I eaten one slice of pizza.

The shift to positive thinking in this realm was a huge turning point for me (aren't they all)!

I realized that exactly because I was overweight, I learned how to eat properly at a much younger age. I became grateful for my eating struggles because it made me learn to eat healthfully. It made me focus on foods that nourished me. Nobody needs a steady diet of artificially flavored, high-sugar, high-fat, processed food that comes in boxes, frozen or from a bakery. The thought of cheese oozing and melting out of a sandwich started to bring pictures of clogged arteries to my mind, instead of the pleasure I used to associate with it. Cake, cookies, chips, ziti, fatty meats, heavy sauces; all the foods I thought I was being deprived of, brought images of fat, not only on the outside of my body, but clogging my arteries on the inside.

Being overweight gave me this gift. I just changed my mind in how I view the same exact things.

I was judged by my physical size. I guess it was hard for anyone to view me in a favorable light. Salespeople ignored me. I saw them looking at me in disgust. I didn't blame them. I also focused on how large and unappealing I was. I remember the shame I felt when I needed help from a salesperson in a department store and they didn't help me. At first I wasn't sure and then I knew I was being completely ignored. They kept helping other shoppers, waiting on normal size people; making believe I didn't exist.

I started to think differently. Would I judge someone only on how they looked? I had overweight friends and family that I loved dearly. In fact, I didn't even notice they were over-weight because I loved them so much. It didn't matter at all. I was concerned for their health. It had zero bearing on my feelings for them.

I loved them because of who they were; not what they looked like. I loved them because I enjoyed their company, they were there for me when I needed them and for countless other reasons. They had many wonderful attributes I admired. I had to start applying the same mindset when it came to myself! My size had nothing to do with the quality of person I was. I took a piece of paper and folded it in half. On one side, I wrote my negatives. On the other side, I wrote my positive attributes.

This simple exercise taught me I was of great value. I was a loving wife, mother, and friend. I gave of my time and money to important causes. The more I thought about who I was and not what I looked like, the happier I became. Shifting the emphasis to who I was had never been suggested at any diet program I went to. That is a shame.
I was put here on this earth for a reason, and it certainly wasn't to ignore what was good about myself.

Learning to love myself was probably the single, most important cognitive change that I made. I had to know and believe with full conviction that I was worthy of achieving my goal if I was to reach my goal. Focusing on my positives allowed me to start liking myself, leading to self-love.

I used to minimize everything I did well, thinking that if I could do it, so could everyone else. If someone complimented anything, I dismissed it, never believing it to be true.

Then I started to wonder. Maybe they are sincere? Maybe I should believe I deserve the compliment. I started paying attention. Guess what? Oftentimes, I was doing a good job. I did put my makeup on nicely that day. I was a caring mother. I did bring smiles to patients at my weekly volunteer visit to a local rehabilitation center. The meal I cooked for a friend, that just had a baby, was delicious. I began to give myself credit where credit was due.

Feeling good about myself spilled over into believing that I was worth the effort to do, what I needed to do, to become my best self. It wasn't easy to change long-standing habits or long-standing beliefs and thoughts, but I started being good to myself. It was okay for me not to jump the moment my name was called. I could finish what I was doing. I could pay the babysitter for an extra half hour, so I would not have to rush through my errands. When that tiny voice, "Who do you think you are?" sneaked in, I immediately squashed it.

Wonderful things began to happen when I started learning to love myself. The more I continued to acknowledge myself, the more I naturally fell into behavior patterns that supported my positive mindset. For example, one night as I was falling asleep I made a mental list of all the things I had to do the next day. My thoughts went something like this, "I know unequivocally that I will definitely not have time to exercise tomorrow. Not possible at all. Simply zero time to schedule that in."

I woke up the next morning and put on my exercise clothes. Huh??? I thought I didn't have time! I went on the elliptical and sweated up a storm. I felt great. I even threw some cauliflower into a pot to steam while I was exercising. I showered and got dressed and went about my day feeling exhilarated. The addition of the cauliflower to my dinner really filled me up and satisfied me.

How did that happen? It happened because I continued to love myself, compliment myself and accept compliments from others. This played a significant role in creating healthy self-esteem. I continually worked on these positive mindsets because they did not come naturally to me. The more I did, the more frequently I lived in a way congruent with those loving messages.

I changed my mind to believe I was worthy of loving myself and accepting love from others. I loved myself enough to stop eating foods that destroyed my beauty and my health. I talked myself into becoming someone that would never mindlessly indulge in food again.

When I finally loved myself enough, I was able to forgive myself for past mistakes. Forgiving myself naturally led to forgiving others, too. I wrote down every single memory that haunted me and every harmful experience that I shoved under layers of fat. I dredged up every buried, uncomfortable thought that I hadn't dealt with. I wrote down every single person I thought I may have harmed. I personally needed to remember and release it all. I could not let these memories weigh me down, figuratively and literally.

Forgiving others can take years but was probably one of the most freeing, amazing things I did for myself! Most of the time, I was the one suffering when not being able to forgive. I was only hurting myself. I learned that most of the time, they didn't even mean to hurt me. Even if they did, I had to learn to say, "Who cares?" In this world, not every single person will like you or will agree with you. That is what makes the world go round. When I realized I was the one that had to change and I was the one that needed a stronger attitude to protect myself, then things began to improve. Waiting for others to change, to speak more nicely to me, to behave better towards me... well, I would probably still be waiting. I was the one that let go of the harmful comments or even obvious attacks. When I dismissed them, I was the one that benefitted. Not giving credence to negativity made my life so much easier.

You don't have to go out and buy ten books on how to forgive. You don't have to research a million articles. Forgiveness, like most everything else, starts in your mind. In some circumstances, I actually called a few people I thought I may have unintentionally harmed. My anxiety before the call was almost unbearable. To my delight and utter surprise, every single friend that I called had the same exact reaction. "What are you talking about? You never upset me!" Here I had been blaming myself for nothing.

I moved forward with promising myself to always face situations straight on. If, at any given moment, I felt like I might have said or done something wrong, I asked immediately. I did not let anything build up. This kept my mind uncluttered. I no longer had to walk around asking, "Did I just say or do the wrong thing?" I inquired on the spot. I didn't leave room for uncertainty in my life.

I looked to everyone else for advice. I looked to everyone else for the answers. Yet, all along, the only one that had the answers that were best for me - was myself. I was the one that needed to take a long, hard look in the mirror and recognize what was not working in my life. I was the one that needed to face what needed to be fixed, changed, improved and altered. I was the one that had to determine which beliefs, thoughts and mindsets did not work in my favor. No one could do that for me. I was in charge of my life and in charge of my own health and wellbeing. I no longer needed someone else to weigh me. I no longer needed to pay someone to put me on a scale. I needed to turn inward. I needed to pay attention to the voice inside of myself and listen to what it was saying.

Don't get me wrong. We still need websites to learn nutritional information to help design an individual food plan, to find healthy recipes and to read about success stories for encouragement. Friends can help make sure the view we see of ourselves is honest. They are great to turn to when needing to talk things through. Know thyself - the support of a trusted therapist, health coach or any form of support you choose can also be very beneficial. You may decide to go to a weight loss center that will allow you to create a personalized food plan; someone to hold your hand through the process. But ultimately, the conversation has to be initiated and ended by you. The more you are involved in creating your goals, steps, and food plan - the greater your chance for success.

I began looking inside myself to figure out what I had to resolve, manage or fix. All the answers had been inside me all along. I just never knew before where to look. The old me, the one that kept me fat, loved playing martyr. I did not know how to create balance in my life. It certainly was not a conscious thing. I had no idea I was operating in that mode. Reflecting back and writing this book turned into a healing process for me. As I dredge up old memories, I uncover more and more memories of what I did to improve myself that in turn improved my life.

A big mistake I made was that I pushed myself to the point of exhaustion and overwhelm. Why did I do this? I did it in search of attention of love. I wrongly thought that the more I did for everyone, the more they would love me. In fact, everything I did for myself was probably because it would also benefit others at the same time.

Before I figured this out, I had this crazy mindset that if I took care of myself for one moment, I was taking care of others one moment less. If I took care of myself for two minutes, I was taking two minutes away from taking care of my family. If I took care of myself for ten minutes, maybe the house would fall down! When my parents came for the weekend, I would stay up crazy late to pour over new menus to make amazing food to please them. I would make sure the sheets were washed and fresh before they were put on their beds. Every holiday, I agonized over making sure that every family member was included and that we made great plans. I could go on and on. But the point is, I remember thinking, "Exercise? Me? Exercise? And take that time away from taking care of my family?" I thought it was selfish. I was so wrong.

I had to learn that taking care of myself is actually taking care of my family! I was so high-strung and on-edge, I could not possibly have been easy to live with. I made myself so busy, that I never relaxed. I was trained to think that if I was happy, that there must be something wrong with that picture. Included in this warped mindset was never knowing how to say, "No." I had been raised as the good girl. Good girls never said no. I always said yes, even when I wanted to say no. I remember trying to make sure I didn't ruffle anyone's feathers. Learning to say no was one of the hardest changes I made. So many of the changes I made are so important. With each one I want to say, "This is the most important thing that I had to change." Learning to say no was huge for me. In fact, my advice to clients is to learn when to say no. Not only is it okay to do so, they are also healing themselves. Obviously, if you can help someone or do a favor, you should! But if you can't, you are allowed to decline.
Now this was the most important thing I had to learn when saying no - to never give an excuse.
When I gave an excuse, it just set me up for a rebuttal. "Of course I understand how stressed you are with work and the kids, but this won't take as much time as you think. I'll help you fit it in." Giving an excuse always weakened my resolve when saying no, because the person asking always had a better reason for me to give in, than I had a reason to decline. Now I simply say, "I would love to but that does not fit into my schedule at this time. Thanks for thinking of me." Of course, when I can, I graciously say, "Yes, I'd love to!"

The lengths I went to for others were completely unnecessary. All I did was dig myself deeper into a bottomless pit. When I did things overboard, I wonder if I actually pushed away those same people whose love and attention I was seeking. Maybe I was coming across desperate and who'd want to love someone like that? Who wants a friend that is harried and stressed? Who wants a mother that is so exhausted that she falls asleep before her head hits the pillow at night? Did my children really need me to completely organize the messy playroom before I allowed myself to go to bed?

I probably would have received much more of what I was thirsty for, if I had been more relaxed. I would have been more fun to be with.

Taking care of myself enabled me to take care of others better. "Just me" time was okay. More than okay! It was necessary for my recovery from food addiction. I got more love and attention from others when I began to have regard for myself. Honoring my time and my needs made me like myself. The more I liked myself, the more I gave off those vibes to others. The more I smiled and relaxed, the more pleasurable it was to connect with me. Taking care of myself, and loving myself, was the best thing I did for my family and friends. As I've mentioned earlier, happiness is contagious!

My recovery from food addiction was aided by creating balance, by deciding what really had to get done, what would be nice if I got it done and what wasn't necessary at all. I had to adjust my thinking to normal. I had to realize I counted and I was important, too.

Living my life on the above cognitive changes has been magical. With my mind "cleaned up," I started to think clearly. My new thoughts were making it much easier to lose weight. They went more like this: *"But...* when you really think about it, Rivka – would you trade your emotional peace of mind for a piece of chocolate cake? Would you give up love and attention for going to the kitchen to scarf down ice cream? Does eating everything you crave make you happy or miserable? Pay attention! Wake up! When you really stop, become aware, and think about the downsides of overeating, would you continue to stuff your face? Would you sacrifice your health, your ability to be presentable when going for a job interview, enjoyment shopping for new clothes and viewing yourself in a dressing room mirror, being confident wherever you are; would you trade any of this for the momentary pleasure of food?"

I worked through my issues, stayed focused and forged ahead. I never gave up. I tried and failed over and over again for decades before I had success. If I could finally do it, you can, too!

Chapter
~ 5 ~

"Write Your Own Story"

1. Write down which cognitive changes you need to make to achieve lasting weight loss?

2. Do you play the victim? If so, how can you stop?

3. Make a list of the wonderful and positive things you do for yourself and others.

4. Do you love yourself? If not, how will you learn to love yourself?

5. Is it possible to forgive yourself and others?

6. Look inside yourself for answers.

7. What issues do you need to address?

8. How will you create balance and boundaries in your life?

Chapter
~ 6 ~

Dealing with Hunger

~ Strategies to Overcome Hunger ~

Yes, my physical body is hungry. My stomach is growling. I haven't eaten in two hours and I really and truly feel a sudden, intense desire to eat. "I want food and I want it now," is happening here. "I don't think I will survive another moment if I don't get my hands on some food."

Is something beyond physical hunger going on here that needs further explanation? Has the desire to eat ever hit so strongly that you can't pay attention to whatever else you were doing? That's because there are many levels and layers to hunger. Yes, truly and simply, you may be only physically hungry. Personally speaking, that was not what was driving my intense, sudden desires to eat.

I needed to inspect, understand and unravel this feeling of hunger. For me, it was much more than physical hunger. My entire being would get hungry. My soul was hungry. I felt empty and needed to be filled. When hunger would strike, yikes, I was reduced to lower-than-childlike instincts. I needed immediate satisfaction. I went to an infantile level. I reacted with anxiousness and desperation when those first barely imperceptible signals of hunger arose.

There. I've revealed it. My big secret is out. "I want to eat, and I want to eat now!" I was like the bull charging into the ring, albeit I was "charging" to my fridge or pantry.
My hunger had many disguises. Clever little back doors tricked me into thinking I needed to eat. Otherwise, I may become malnourished.

What is hunger? The definition is "A strong desire or need for food. The discomfort, weakness, or pain caused by a prolonged lack of food. A strong desire or craving, as for affection."

Interesting, very interesting! This definition hit home for me. I may have imagined discomfort when hunger would strike. I may have imagined weakness or pain. However, that really wasn't possible because I rarely experienced a "prolonged lack of food!" The "strong desire or craving, as for affection" - now that is something I could relate to! Where did that leave me? I would venture a guess that very early on, I totally messed up my hunger signals of "I need to eat" from "I need to fill my emptiness."

It was imperative for me to learn to distinguish physical hunger from emotional hunger if I was to have any success. I learned to listen to my body's signals. If I felt hunger, but it didn't make sense that I should be hungry, I paid attention to what was going on right before the desire to eat started.
I set out to uncover what just occurred and what triggered the hunger sensation by allotting a short period of time to resolving this mystery. Was I truly feeling physically hungry, growling stomach and all, when I just experienced an emotionally upsetting event? Was I just thinking that I was dissatisfied or frustrated with myself? Misinterpreted feelings

71

of physical hunger could even arise out of boredom. Setting a specific amount of time, promising myself that I wouldn't automatically eat when the first physical sensations of hunger arose, allowed me to figure out what was truly going on.

Here are some of the strategies I found that worked best to help me stop eating on "automatic pilot." I kept an "Activities List" everywhere. I posted them in my bedroom, on my cell phone, on my computer, and into the insides of my kitchen cabinets. Everywhere! I had to break the cycle of immediately eating with the first hunger pang. Instead of eating, I did an activity from my list. My "Activities List" looked like this:

~ Run, don't walk and get out of kitchen
~ Drink a glass of water
~ Read motivating weight-loss stories
~ Review reasons I want to lose weight
~ Leave house for a few minutes
~ Call a friend
~ Play piano
~ Check my email
~ Polish my nails
~ Pick up a cookbook to find healthy recipes
~ Run up and down the staircase
~ Do jumping jacks

After I did an activity, which distanced my mind from food, I was able to think more clearly. I could then think about which foods I was craving. I began to notice a pattern.
When I craved cookies, cake, sugar-laden foods, and high-fat foods, I realized more often than not, that I was either tired, upset with myself or with someone else, frustrated, lonely,

72

bored or I had neglected my own needs. This helped me understand what caused me to believe I was hungry. I was hungry for some rest, a friend's ear for advice, some fun or doing something for myself. This hunger was an indication of an emotionally-based urge to eat. When I started thinking salad, fruit or a tuna sandwich, the hunger usually turned out to be physical. When I was truly hungry, I craved food.

Another reason I felt hungry was because I was not eating enough carbohydrates. Too many people are on very high protein and fat diets with limited vegetables, fruits and whole grains. This may work for some, as I do believe everyone is different. There is no one right diet for all, but I was frequently not satisfied and was truly hungry too soon after meals. I was severely limiting my healthy carbohydrates. I rarely allowed myself foods like oatmeal, quinoa or fruit. I even limited high-carbohydrate vegetables like carrots and winter squashes. My body was craving the nutrients and fiber from these healthy foods. I was on this vicious cycle for decades. Because high-protein diets were touted as the best and only possible way to lose weight for many years, as I have mentioned earlier, I was most often on that type of diet. For me, that was the worst diet possible. That is precisely why my body cried hunger.

I had to learn the hard way that for me to be satisfied, I needed large portions of salad and vegetables and enough wholesome grains. It makes me sad to remember that many of the diet places I went to, and paid good money, actually restricted me in this way. You may be eating enough calories. You may be eating enough quantity. But the quality of the diet may not be meeting your particular nutritional needs.

If you have stayed away from carbohydrates, even healthy ones, and can't seem to stay satisfied, it may be time to add some sprouted whole-grain bread or some slow-cooked oatmeal to your food plan. There are amazing new products coming out now. I love my black bean pasta. It is literally made out of 92% black beans and 8% water. Those are the ingredients! Adding these foods may help eliminate your hunger. It eliminated mine.

Another addition to satisfying my hunger was adding a wide variety of beans. Once again, I shied away from beans because the labels said they contained carbohydrates. I was listening to all the high-protein hype. Chicken, fish, meat, egg, and cheese had zero carbohydrates. I wrongly chose those foods over beans, fruits and vegetables for decades. Again, a high-protein may be the best diet for you. However, it certainly was not for me. Learn to listen to what *your* body is trying to tell you. Listen closely and you will get all the right answers.

I also totally eliminated root vegetables because I was, once again, incorrectly told that they are fattening and have too many carbohydrates. I am not saying they are a free-for-all like romaine lettuce, but I think they add a nice variety to a meal and are full of vitamins. Carrots, sweet potatoes, winter squashes, such as acorn and butternut, will satisfy you much longer than a few cups of lettuce and radishes. Adding only half-a-cup of these grounding root vegetables will satisfy you for the long run.
Additionally, I believe I often became hungry because my body was trying to tell me I had a nutritional deficiency. I always craved foods like nuts, beans, avocados, dark leafy greens, and dark chocolate. I could make a joke about the

chocolate here, but seriously, all those foods have magnesium in them. I found out that I had a magnesium deficiency.

I also mistook thirst for hunger. That's why drinking a glass of water was on my activities list. I frequently added organic lemon juice or even some fresh lemon slices. The lemon water helped me distinguish thirst from hunger plus I got a nice dose of vitamin C. Oftentimes, the glass of water completely took away the hunger. It still does.

So I first allotted a short period of time between my hunger craving and eating, got out of the kitchen and then took a drink of water. I spent a few minutes on one of the activities from my list. By then I was able to determine whether I was truly hungry or not. If I was hungry, and it was less than one hour till my next meal, I did not eat. This was a good exercise for me because it taught me that *nothing happened when I went hungry for one hour*. I didn't faint. I didn't pass out. Seriously, I tried it and I am still here. It's okay. It's okay to be hungry sometimes.

Let's now discuss hunger and hormones. When I was younger, much younger, it was really super-hard to distinguish hormonal cravings from physical hunger. Let's just say that a premenstrual or menstrual woman could easily win an eating contest against a whale. At least I could have back in the day. When you know you are a week before your cycle or during that week, I would humbly suggest just talking to yourself, over and over again, as many times as need be, "I am not truly hungry. I am just a crazed female due to an outpouring of bazillions of hormones racing through my body and just because I feel like I can eat an entire chocolate factory, does not mean that I should." Be careful during this time, because if you are anything like I was, this is the time when you're most likely to convince yourself that you are hungry, even when you are not. So shoo those hormonal demons away by completely ignoring them and not giving them any credence, as much as you can.

Another way the mind fools us into thinking we are really hungry, besides hormones, is simply a desire to feel good when we are feeling down. Our brains release feel-good chemical, also called natural opiates including serotonin. Be aware that eating foods high in sugar and carbohydrates releases them and, therefore, improve your mood.

Cravings, whether from a physical, emotional or nutritional source, can indeed be incredibly strong and difficult to overcome. If they weren't, we wouldn't have any problem saying "No" to food. But we do have so much trouble; so much so, that even knowing and saying to ourselves, "I shouldn't be eating this. I want to lose weight so badly. I know my health is in jeopardy. I know I am upset just because my boss yelled at me, but I still want to eat. I am overwhelmed with everything that needs to get done, and I know I am not hungry, but I still want to eat." - we still pick up the food.

Everyone is different, so I will discuss one more strategy that many of my clients find helpful. Even if you determined that you are not hungry, on any level, some people still need that chewing sensation. You may choose to chew on ice chips or sugar-free gum. Others may not need to put anything in their mouth at all and find something to do with their hands. I find it best not to involve my mouth. Seriously. Chewing on anything makes me want to chew even more. Some of you may need to pick up a crochet hook, knitting needle or pen to make a sketch. When your fingers are busy, they can't pick up food. Others may need to use their whole body and do jumping jacks or lift some weights. The point is to find an activity to replace eating. The more you replace responding to that hunger signal with specific activities, the more your brain will register hunger with that activity or activities. Clients have shared great ideas for activities such as prayer, meditation, or phoning a supportive friend. Now the job is to choose which activities work best for *you* – the ones that get you away from food, the ones that break the cycle. The more you do this, the more likely you will do it again in the future.

When you've removed that automatic and instinctual eating from your repertoire, success will come so much sooner and you'll feel great about yourself. I felt like I had literally created new pathways in my brain so that instead of picking up the food, I automatically got busy. When I became in control of my food, I was more in control in my life. Becoming aware of true hunger, and choosing to eat appropriately, had a ripple effect on other areas of my life. I was in control, which led to being that way in general. So choose which activities are most likely to work for you. Choose the ones you can go to easily.

Do not use the excuse I used! I convinced myself that I did not have time and was too busy to fit in an activity. I was sabotaging myself. I was fooling myself. I would make excuses for years that I did not have time to stop what I was doing when it finally dawned on me that I was eating for at least ten, fifteen, twenty minutes or more! I could have spared myself so much misery of being fat if I had taken that time to do an activity instead of stuffing my face.

What if you can't identify the hunger? What if it does not fall into any of these categories? There was something much deeper than physical, emotional or nutritional hunger tugging at me. A space so huge, so cavernous to fill that the word hunger simply wasn't enough. There was a space deep inside me, way deep inside, that was aching. Hunger was not the correct word. It didn't encompass this drive to eat. It fell way too short. There was a yearning, a longing to be satiated that no amount of activities, chewing or food could ever begin to fill.

What was that empty space? What was I desiring? There was a hollowness for a type of connection that I could barely discern. When certain things fell into place, the faint message started to get louder and stronger. My insides were screaming for that space to be filled. I call that space spirituality. Read on and live through the wondrous journey of how bringing spirituality into my life helped fill my hungry soul.

Chapter
~ 6 ~

"Write Your Own Story"

1. Write down how you successfully overcame over-eating when hungry.

2. How do you differentiate between physical and emotional hunger?

3. Create your own list of activities to go to when you get hungry.

4. Is eliminating certain food groups an explanation for unexplained food cravings?

5. Are you hungry for love, hugs, attention or appreciation?

Chapter
~ 7 ~

Spirituality

~ Embracing G-d's Help ~

Sometime during my weight loss journey I met a woman. She truly sparked my delving deeper into G-d and spirituality. It was one of the major remedies in recovering from my addiction to food.

I was having success, but not as much as I could have. I still experienced extremely powerful, unexplainable urges to eat. Being a religious person, I believed that I aligned my life to the will of my Creator. I came to understand that I practiced on a diluted, superficial level. I had a connection but did not realize how tiny it was compared to where it could and should have been.

I decided to learn more about my own religion. I began attending classes, speaking to spiritual leaders and reading many books. The more I learned, the more I became aware and believed that G-d wanted to be personally involved in my life, one-on-one, that He was truly interested in what happened to me and involved at every moment. I then understood that I had a loving G-d that wanted to be in my life and wanted me to be involved in His life, through prayer and speaking to Him even in my own simple language.

I considered myself one of the lucky ones. I was summoned to do more. Had I not been tormented by food, I may never have begun my spiritual journey. Maybe G-d would have tapped on my window through some avenue other than food; I'll never know. I came to understand that being fat led me to unhappiness, which in turn caused me to fall into depression. All this was actually my soul calling, "Hey, wake up! You are not anywhere near where you could and should be in your relationship with G-d!"

Up until this point, I viewed my problems as punishments. I thought I was being punished by this crazy obsession with food. Somehow I began to grasp that this was not G-d's intention, not in the least. He knew me best. He knew that in order to shake me awake to His calling, He had to use this route. Only in hindsight do I see that what I viewed as punishment turned out to be one of the biggest blessings in my life. I realized that I had been given a precious gift. How did I come to acknowledge this fact? Calling the same thing that made me miserable a gift? The answer is actually quite simple.

Had I just been rolling merrily along in my life, I would have stagnated and remained the same in religion and in the way I chose to live everyday life. Had I been happy, without any problems, I would not have become aware of how much richer my religious life could be. I would not have become aware of how much joy and satisfaction I would personally experience, by learning the holy sacred texts of my religion, ultimately bringing me closer to G-d.

In addition to the above, had I not been miserable, maybe I

would not have become an artist. Being an artist was a way of expressing outwards the suppressed feelings I did not understand and could not hold inside. Being an artist was also a way of busying myself with something other than another visit to the refrigerator.

I had no idea that I had been operating on a shallow version of life. I had no idea I could accomplish and become so much more. My food addiction squeezed out parts of myself I would have never discovered had I not been pushed forward by feeling miserable.

Had I not gone through a major self-makeover, I would not have felt the urge to go back to school to become a Life Coach, giving me the tools to help others with their lives. Had I not become a Life Coach, I would not have found out about the health coaching school I attended, enriching my knowledge of nutrition manifold. I sincerely believe this was all divinely orchestrated, starting with my being fat!

Now I had a big bridge to cross. On one side, were my food challenges. On the other side, I had my intense calling for more spirituality. Talk about disparate elements. How do I link those two areas together? How do I connect and involve G-d with my ridiculously embarrassing food binges?

Creating a relationship with G-d took root. An intimate connection truly happened. I learned to thank Him immensely for every single detail. My gratitude list included the most seemingly insignificant things that I used to take for granted. I opened my eyes and began appreciating all the good in my life. Besides thanking G-d, I learned to ask for advice on parenting, marriage, relationships; the gamut! This came easily to me. But talk to Him about donuts and bagels? Nonsense.

But something kept tapping at my consciousness. I started understanding that if G-d was with me in my life, I had to allow Him to help me with this challenge, too. I decided to ask for His guidance when the overwhelming crazies to binge set in. Just like I would go to G-d and beseech His help in other areas of my life, I figured, "Why not? Give it a whirl." I already submitted to attaching myself to Him in every other arena of my life, and, so too, I would now try getting advice and guidance with my food problems. The more I thought about it, the more I was embarrassed at the thought of using and abusing food in the way that I did, as if He didn't already know. He certainly did not create food for me to harm myself with. He created food for survival. I was doing the exact opposite with the food I was blessed with. I was killing myself with it. Talk about a light bulb moment. Not only did the light bulb light up, but sirens, bells, and whistles sounded just to make sure I got the message.

I accepted that I could not do this on my own. I could not trust myself when it came to making the best choices, especially when the tough times got going. So that was the easy part; telling myself that I should go to Him for advice. The hard part was at that actual moment of choice - I had to make it a habit to go immediately to G-d and ask for help, rather than going to food for my "fix."

When I used to feel a binge coming, the anxiety would start rumbling up inside me. Many times it began, seemingly without any cause, and with immense anxiety and intensity. I would head straight to the fridge. At that moment, I had to choose between comfort from G-d or comfort from food. Choosing comfort from G-d became a necessary ingredient for my being able to stay away from the food. As small as it may seem in the grand scheme of life's challenges, I believe that I get points every single time I do not binge. I believe that not only are we wired differently and genetically as to how our brains function, I believe we are wired differently spiritually. When I began to believe that this was a God-given challenge, I delved right in. The spirituality or religious gene, whatever you want to label it, was definitely there and growing stronger every day.

For sure, I wanted to lose weight. For sure, I wanted to go to a normal clothing store. For sure, I wanted to be healthy. This, however, put losing weight onto a much higher playing field. If this was a God-given challenge, then He certainly would help get me out of it. Would this alone have worked? I do not believe so. I had to work on myself enough, to get to this point, where I was aware enough to open myself up to His help. In the early stages of my "brain fog," I doubt I could have achieved this.

I did this often, with G-d's presence very palpable. Through the years, the habit of not going to the food, has allowed Him to recede. This is not a conscious activity at this point but I believe He knows that I can now be on my own, with Him in the wings if I need Him again. I still speak to Him every day but I include a lot more now than "food" talk.

Here's a case in point. I was in a terrible car accident. I didn't realize I turned onto the railroad tracks instead of the street (both street lamps were out, the street I was turning from and the street I was turning onto). My car stopped and seemed stuck. I couldn't go forward. I couldn't go in reverse. It was so dark that I didn't have a clue why I couldn't move my car. The next moment, the entire front-end of my three-week old car was ablaze in flames. I realized I was on the railroad tracks and thought, "I have to get out of this car. A train could come!"

I miraculously came out unscathed. The car was in the shop for three weeks. The anxiety level was high. I was trembling from the experience. My emotions were high from all the flashing lights, policemen, firemen, and bystanders. When I got home, I called a friend for some well-needed support. The friend brought a plate of jelly donuts. I know it was her way of saying, "I don't know what to do but here, eat these, you'll feel better."

When my friend left, I stared at the jelly donuts. I took the plate from the living room to the kitchen. I said to myself, "Look what you've been through. Of course, you can have the jelly donuts." But I remembered that G-d would be much more comforting to me than a jelly donut. I asked Him to hold my hand and remove the desire for the donuts. The same God that saved my life on the railroad tracks could certainly fill this request.

It worked. I felt G-d's support at that moment. I overcame my strong urges to eat the donuts. I couldn't believe it. The urges that were so strong to eat the them melted away as I felt myself being ensconced in warmth from G-d.

I picked up the plate of donuts, walked to the garbage, and threw them away. He saved me from the jelly donuts, too.

Now I can say, "Thank You for my food challenges and insanity with food, because they brought me closer to You."

Knowing that G-d has my back and knowing He wants me healthy continues to be a huge part of my going forward and being able to stop going to food for comfort.

Instead of going to food, I go to Him. Knowing that He is listening and knowing that He cares for my health, keeps me away from abusing food and from abusing myself.

Chapter
~ 7 ~

"Write Your Own Story"

1. Are you tapped into G-d, spirituality, something or someone other than yourself?

2. Do you consider that there is a force greater than yourself?

3. Ponder these deep thoughts and see who you can go to for help.

Chapter
~ 8 ~

Food Changes for Success

~ Quality of Food Does Matter ~

I changed what I ate. Big time. Major. I did a huge pantry and fridge makeover. Why? I did not have real food in my house. I was the typical kid of the 50's and 60's growing up during the explosion of frozen TV dinners, convenience food and boxed cookies, snacks and junk foods. They made life easy. They made life delicious. Who ever thought, "But is it good for me?"

Here is the reality. Only real food truly satisfies. Couple this with the fact that eating real food also revved up my metabolism, giving me a winning combination. What is real food? As you read this chapter, you will begin to understand. There are no miracle drugs, combinations of foods, elimination of food groups, time of day to eat, time of day to not eat, food combining or eating for your body type that will help you lose weight long-term. When I eliminated categories of real foods, I ultimately craved them. I am referring to healthy food groups such as fruits, grains, nuts, protein, etc. Many books told me there is too much sugar in fruit and too many carbohydrates in grains. Unless you have some medical reason to cut out certain foods, the best diet is to eat what is found in nature.

This is what real food is all about. Yes, if G-d made it, if nature made it, if the universe created it – those foods became the mainstay of my diet.

Companies began to remove the healthy outer husks of brown rice turning it into white rice that can boil in a minute. Potato chips started being made from potato starch or potato flour. What happened to real sliced potatoes? How are children's snacks the colors red, yellow, pink and blue? Ever wonder why food in bags and boxes on supermarket shelves last so long? Maybe we should all start paying attention.

The unprocessed, as close to nature as possible foods, are the ones I began to focus on. Those are the foods that filled my plate. By eating those nutrient dense foods, portion control became so much easier. Real foods satisfy. When I was more satisfied, I did not need a measuring cup to tell me how much to eat.

I was completely wrong thinking low-calorie foods had little nutritional value. I figured there was some type of correlation between calories and nutrient content. I thought if a food had more calories, logic would follow that it would have more vitamins and minerals. I was wrong. This is simply not true!
For example, I always knew that celery had very few calories. Therefore, I assumed it had very little nutritional value. The same with cucumbers; even the color "told" me that these vegetables were devoid of nutrients. Definitely not true! These foods provide amazing health benefits!

Listen to the amazing power of the celery stick. It's almost too good to be true but celery provides vitamin K, folate, potassium, manganese, vitamin B2, copper, vitamin C, vitamin B6, phosphorus, magnesium, calcium and vitamin A. What are the health benefits of eating celery? What ailments can celery naturally cure? Celery has been shown to reduce high blood pressure, prevent cancer, lower cholesterol and promote overall health. All these benefits with hardly any calories. Why would I eat a donut? Why would I eat a pretzel or potato chip? I had to drill into my head that no amount of food could outweigh my desire to be healthy. Guess what? I actually love the way celery tastes now. Sometimes I spread a little almond butter on it, too.

It's good to have fruit! I eat all varieties of berries, all kinds of apples, oranges, and melons. I never went to any diet center that allowed me to eat more than one fruit for a snack and certainly never more than two a day.

I just took a mid-morning break from writing a few minutes ago. I ate a kiwi, an orange, some cashews and a few dates with a cup of tea. Back in the day, I would have scolded myself. I would have thought I was not in control. I would have thought I ate too much. I had never been to a diet center or diet doctor that allowed me to eat *that* much for a snack.

When I thought about what I wanted to snack on, I was totally in control. It was more than I normally have but I was hungrier than usual. I intuitively ate a smaller lunch. Some steamed cauliflower with quinoa and pumpkin seeds sprinkled on top. I enjoyed my larger than usual snack, while instinctively eating a smaller lunch. I have never weighed less in my life. It has become automatic to create a healthy balance of food across the course of each day by including fruits, vegetables, fats, nuts, seeds, whole grains, and protein. How do I do this? I listen to myself. I pay attention by consciously stopping and asking, "What am I in the mood for?"

You need to experiment and see what works for *you*. There are exceptions to every rule. Some people are better off staying away from eating in-between meals completely. Some should definitely have a snack. Some people need to eliminate even healthy whole grains if they contain gluten. Just because your friend eliminated gluten and feels better does not mean you should, too. If your friend eliminated white flour and sugar, then I'd say be a "copycat." Nobody needs to eat those.

Are there certain percentages of foods that should be eaten each day? Again, everyone is different. If you walk into a food program that hands you a list of foods, and they eliminate carrots and tomatoes, run the other way. If they tell you to take out scales and measuring cups, run the other way. If they give the same exact plan to everyone that comes into their office, without even going over your medical history, food preferences and lifestyle, run the other way. They do not know you! How could they possibly advise how you should eat? Do they know your likes and dislikes? Do they know what you enjoy eating? A place well worth spending your money is where they create an individualized menu for *you* and provide support to keep up your commitment.

You are probably thinking, at this very moment, "Not weigh and measure?" Let me share a startling revelation with you. Let's say that now you are eating three slices of pizza for dinner. If you eat two slices of pizza, you reduced your calories by a third. Eating more than one bagel? I certainly did. I ate two, three and even four bagels at a meal. Had I eaten one bagel, I would have been able to prevent myself from so much misery and suffering. Do you really need to be told to eat one bagel, and preferably a whole wheat or pumpernickel bagel? One bagel has a quarter the calories of eating four bagels. Hmmm, and I was not a math major. Half a bagel has half the calories than a whole bagel. Wow! Eating half a cow at dinner? Try one steak or a few slices of meat. Try a quarter of a chicken instead of a half. Slice your usual portion in half and you will have - you guessed it, you genius! You have half the calories! Starting to get the picture? Starting to see why I abhor scales and measuring cups? Start being honest with yourself. Look at your plate. If you really don't have a clue what a normal portion should be, that's ok. Start with eating less. Period. Begin by taking off a third of your usual portion. Maybe you need to cut the meal in half? Start paying attention to your body and your needs.

Only real food is truly physically satiating. This is no surprise! When you eat empty calories that come in a box, with zero nutrition and no fiber, of course, you will not be satisfied and will go back again and again. Fruits, vegetables, and beans have fiber. Fiber is what gives us that full feeling. The fiber from the food expands with the liquids in our bodies to create the sensation that we have had enough.

I believe that the Nutrition Fact label has done almost more harm than good. Yes, it is great to know how much sodium is in a food. It is helpful to know how much protein. However, I became aware that food companies are very savvy. Just because a label states that a boxed food has fiber, please become an educated consumer, and don't believe everything you read. I noticed this claim on the front of a sugary, chocolate-flavored children's cereal, "A good source of fiber."

Really? Sugar and chocolate, artificial coloring, and artificial flavor, have fiber? Upon further inspection, I read this ingredient, "poly-dextrose." Does that grow on a farm? Is that picked from a tree? I was curious so I looked it up on the Internet. Seems that it is a newfangled fiber additive, creating the illusion that this cereal is actually good for your kids, providing them with a full day's fiber! Are we sprayed with invisible "stupid spray" when entering a supermarket, and then sprayed with "un-stupid spray" when we leave? Do I really need a Nutrition Fact Label to tell me that a child would have more fiber eating a bowl of oatmeal and an orange for breakfast? Do I really need a Nutrition Fact label to tell me the nutrition information on boxed children's cereals? Do I believe that any of them are in any shape, manner or form, good for them? I asked the owner of my supermarket to stop spraying me with "stupid spray." Now I know that none of them are good for my grandchildren.

Seriously, the general population was much healthier and slimmer before Nutrition Fact labels ever existed. In fact, most of the food I eat now does not even come with a Nutrition Fact label. The less you eat foods that come in a box or a package, the slimmer you will be. The less take-out food you buy, the healthier you will be. The more you cook your own food, the better for you and your entire family. Let me share a great story that recently happened to me. I went to visit a friend that had a knee replacement. She said, "Oh, great. I have another friend coming soon that is in the food industry." I guess being a health and weight loss coach included me in the "food industry." Her lovely friend joined us soon thereafter. Here was her reply, when I inquired what her job entails, "We test food to see the minimal amount of sugar we can add to create a desire to go back for more." I wish I had a video camera rolling on me at that moment. I wish you could have seen my facial expression upon hearing these words. I had to stop myself from putting my hands around her throat and shake her, while screaming, "Are you out of your mind?" I guess a paycheck is a paycheck.

The first time I heard about this I was like, "Nah, nobody would go that low." Unfortunately, this is what is happening in our society. Read the ingredients. Almost every single food today has some kind of sugar added, and unnecessarily I may add. So do you think we are both involved in the same "food industry?"

Still find food that comes in a box appealing? Oh, and one more side point about food with Nutrition Fact labels. Where is the percentage for sugar? Ever notice that is missing? Interesting. Think they forgot to add the percentage of sugar? I'm curious as to why this is omitted.

I look back and think, "Did I really think an ounce of pretzels would nourish and satisfy me the same as an apple?" Ridiculous. But the plan that was handed to me said I could have an ounce of pretzels for a snack. Don't get me wrong, I am not saying you can never have pretzels, but honestly, the way I eat now, I rarely eat them because they do not have any nutritional value. If I want something crunchy, I'll eat raw jicama or pepper strips.

There is an old saying, "Eat breakfast like a king, lunch like a prince and dinner like a pauper." Try to eat this way. Try having a larger breakfast and lunch that include your higher-calorie foods, and a light dinner. A benefit to eating a light dinner is sleeping better. I find I sleep best when my dinner is light and I don't have an evening snack.

Try viewing your whole day's meals and snacks. For example, if you ate whole grains at breakfast and lunch, skip them at dinner. You can still have an incredibly filling meal. Have vegetable soup, a salad with some protein and a fruit for dessert. This will become second nature. If you know you are going out for a special dinner, it's okay to enjoy a larger meal once in awhile, but then do cut back on breakfast and lunch that day.

Here's the best advice – do not overeat! I recently saw a poster that read, "It's the food stupid." I *was* stupid. Did I really need to be a rocket scientist to figure out that I was overeating? Yes, my weight loss slowed down as I got closer to my goal weight but enough of the right exercise ultimately kept the scale moving downwards.

Every overweight person weighs too much because they eat too much food and usually the wrong foods (with rare exception), coupled with a lack of physical activity. Do you really need anyone to tell you that you need to eat less? Listen, I am one of you – I have been blessed to now be living in a much smaller body but my mind is still wired exactly like yours. I went to doctors and diet centers and sincerely exclaimed at my first visits, "But I do not eat that much!" I truly believed what I said. Yes, on the days I actually dieted, or starved myself, I didn't eat that much. However, the diet days certainly didn't outweigh the binge days by any stretch.

More than twenty-five years ago, I spent three hundred dollars to go to a famous Park Avenue diet doctor. He basically told me one thing. Keep a food journal. I was in a state of denial when it came to admitting how much food I ate. I have brilliant clients that are extremely successful in every other area of their lives, they can remember the most minute details for work, come up with brilliant solutions for their companies but blank out completely when it comes to remembering just how much they ate that day. I did the same thing. I "blanked out" the bingeing.

So if you truly believe you do not overeat and that you are the victim of a poor metabolism, try keeping a journal. Write down every single morsel that you put into your mouth. If you are overweight, and you truly think you don't eat enough to be overweight, keeping a journal may make you realize that you eat a lot more than you thought you did. I had to journal my food. It showed me that I was eating a lot more than I thought I was. Do not forget to jot down even what you drink. Do not forget anything. It's for your own good. So please be kind to yourself. Adjust your portions. Try not eating as frequently as you used to. See what works for you, so that the scale will move downwards.

So does the quality of food really matter? Yes! For me, it mattered so much. My weight loss was still very slow and I was still struggling. When I started paying attention to the quality of my food, my weight loss began to accelerate. What do I mean by the quality? The quality of the food or "clean" eating definitely made a difference. When I did research to see if anything supported what I was experiencing, I found a lot! The body simply cannot function optimally when bombarded with chemicals and artificial ingredients. Our bodies are designed to keep us healthy, but the body can do only so much. When it is trying to figure out, "Hey, what's dye #4 and how do I process this toxic chemical and that toxic pesticide?" it is so busy using its resources to keep us well that is has no energy left, so to speak, to aid your metabolism. When you are eating "clean" your body's basic functioning can increase by not diverting energies to other areas, like ridding itself of toxicity. When eating clean, your metabolism can kick in. I experienced this and so can you.

When I became aware that our crops are sprayed with chemicals and pesticides, I was really surprised. Where have I been? How come I wasn't informed? Animals are being injected with bovine growth hormone and who knows what else, to fatten them up and increase production and therefore sales. Cows, for example, are injected with chemicals for the purpose of increasing milk production. Is anyone else thinking, "Nice. Zero regulations on how artificially altered our foods have become but no one told us?"

So become aware and try as best you can to ask questions. Become an informed consumer. The heads of almost every department in my local supermarket know me by name. I asked for each one's cell phone number. I call to make sure they have what I want in stock. I call or text the produce guy, "Any organic broccoli or organic romaine today?" If yes, I ask him to please put some aside for me. Ahead of time, I email the butcher for an order of organic chicken. When I find out about new, organic products, I ask them to carry it and if their distributor can get it, it's on the shelf within a short time. If you need any assistance in your local supermarket, just ask!

Other ingredients I stay away from are artificial coloring, artificial flavoring, artificial sweeteners, genetically modified foods, monosodium glutamate, sugar, propellants and ingredients I can't pronounce (99% of the time it's stuff we should not be eating). If you can't pronounce it, don't buy it. Did you notice propellants? Look at the ingredients for any of the zero-calorie oil sprays; they all have propellants. I'd rather use a tablespoon of real oil.

Organic anyone? Why do people look at me like I am wearing bell-bottom jeans and a mandarin-collared shirt when I tell them I eat organic? Why do I have to convince and demonstrate the truth that organic is merely what we ate in past generations? Why do we have to label foods organic? Why shouldn't it be that foods with harmful and unnatural ingredients should be labeled? Why shouldn't they have to put on their labels: "Warning! This modified food has pesticides, the percentage of sugar in this food is more than your ancestors ate in a month, and food coloring dye #3 and #4 are in here, too."

Why don't those labels read, "Do you know what you are feeding your child?" Or how about, "Do you know that studies have shown that monosodium glutamate causes brain cell damage in babies and children?"

I am tired of trying to prove to friends and family that they need to read the ingredient labels to ascertain if it's really food they are eating. How come I feel like the odd one out because I want to only buy organic fruits and vegetables.

How come I feel like the "hippie" of our times not wanting to consume fruits and vegetables sprayed with pesticides. How come I'm the weirdo because I travel to farmer's markets and health food stores for clean food.

But here's a great story. I had guests for a meal. Of course, somehow the conversation always turns to, "Rivka only buys organic." Yes, I paid more to feed you organic, not just my family. Yes, the vegetables, fruits, and chicken you are eating are all organic.

My friends' husband, while rolling his eyes, said to me, "You think my grandparents ate organic?"

He gave me the perfect setup for my reply! I was able to significantly turn around his thinking with one short explanation. "Exactly. Eating organic is what your grand-parents ate." I told him the food did not have to be labeled organic because all food was naturally organic. Their food was not sprayed with chemicals and pesticides. They used nature to protect vegetables on farms. They knew that planting certain plants around particular vegetables would ward off bugs.
I literally saw the "Aha" moment on his face. I literally saw a light bulb go off in his brain! He got it! He looked at me and said, "Now I understand. You are right."

Incredible when you start to pay attention. Chances are that most of the food you are purchasing is not real food and has been processed, altered or preserved in some way that strips vital minerals, nutrients and fiber.

When I starting eating real food, the theory of calorie in, calorie out, just seemed to disappear. I strongly encourage you to not be afraid of the calories from any healthy, real food. I do not have a clue how many calories I eat per day but I have an interesting story to tell you about my husband. He's tall, slim and doesn't have to watch his weight. Yep, that's the guy I married. Even though he was slim, he ate tons of junk - donuts, pastries, chips and red meat. I cooked mostly vegetarian for my family, limiting my children's snacks to mostly fruits and vegetables (they weren't happy back in the day but now as adults they are grateful.) He still did his own thing. For many years I tried to get him to eat healthier but to no avail. He snacked on bags, and I mean bags, of chocolate chips.

Recently, we watched several movies about the connection nowadays between food and the increase in many illnesses. All of a sudden, he stopped eating his chocolate chips. When I noticed, I asked him how he managed to give up a lifelong habit cold-turkey. How could he go from snacking all day on chocolate chips to not eating any? He laughed and replied, "I replaced the chocolate chips with bags of nuts. The movies we watched really changed my mind."
"Nuts?" you might ask. Don't nuts have a bazzilion calories for a tiny amount. Yes, they do. That is just my point. We calculated that my husband added about 7,500 calories every week or so to his diet. The chocolate chips had way fewer calories than the nuts. A funny thing happened. He was not trying to lose weight. He did not need to lose weight. He dropped four and a half pounds in the first few weeks. Calories in – calories out? I don't think so. My husband and I alone are obviously not scientific evidence for proving this, but as I wrote in my introduction, I am sharing my story.

I am telling you what I did to lose weight and to easily maintain my weight loss. I eat half an avocado almost every day. I put olive oil or avocado oil on my salads; no measuring, just a quick pour straight from the bottle. Most of the diets I was given didn't allow avocados and restricted me to tiny amounts of oil, if any. My non-stick pans went in the garbage and I now use oil when I cook. I, too, eat at least half-a-cup of nuts per day, if not more, and my weight stays the same. If you add up those calories, plus the rest of my food, I now must be eating twice the calories I ate when I was much heavier.

When it comes to food, nourishing your body is what it is all about. It thanks you by performing well. When you really think about it, it's like a car. Would you put cheap gas in your car? Would you put in anything other than real gas in your car? If someone came over to you and said, "Hey, I've got this artificial stuff but it's half the price of gasoline," would you buy it? Of course not. If you did succumb to the cheaper price, your car would let you know by not running well or by not running at all. Our bodies are no different. Fuel it up with calories that count. It will give back by performing optimally for your health and your metabolism.

Another important factor in losing weight is enjoying all the food you eat. As I already mentioned, I remember for years and years eating plain hard-boiled eggs because that was supposed to make you lose weight. I remember eating grapefruit after grapefruit because that was supposed to make you lose weight. The problem was I didn't like plain hard-boiled eggs, but that is what I was told to eat to lose weight. I didn't like grapefruit! "Can I eat an orange," I'd ask. "No," was the answer, if I wanted to lose weight. Grapefruits will burn off the fat. Not an orange. And so, I listened. But the result was that I never felt satisfied. I ate what I thought I was supposed to eat to lose weight. I followed the breakfast, lunch and dinner guidelines of countless diet center and diet books to a "t." I was strict. I was perfect. The problem was I didn't like the taste of the foods I was eating. In order to feel satisfied, I needed my food to be delicious. Feeling satisfied is an important factor in keeping yourself from overeating. Feeling satisfied is very different from feeling full. We can feel satisfied and not feel full. In fact, if you feel full, you most definitely overate!

You need to recognize your own taste buds and not listen to what someone else tells you to eat. You need to organize your meals in such a way that you are completely satisfied, having foods from a wide variety of categories.

The color of different foods is an easy guide to help you fill your nutritional needs. Think about it. The more colorful your plate, the easier it is to know that you are eating a good variety of foods and, therefore, a good range of vitamins. When you think of orange foods, think mangos, sweet potatoes, nectarines, oranges, orange bell peppers and apricots. Yellow would include yellow peppers, corn, lemons and spaghetti squash. Red foods are apples, cherries, kidney beans, radishes, tomatoes and strawberries. White foods are bean dips, hummus, legumes, onions, shallots, nuts, chicken and fish. Green foods, my favorites, are broccoli, chard, cucumbers, string beans, lettuces, olives, spinach, celery, kale and cabbage. Last but not least are the purple and blue foods. Think blueberries, purple kale, black rice, purple potatoes, grapes, eggplant and plums. See how easy eating well can be when using color? When eating a variety of colors, you cover a lot of different vitamins and minerals because you are eating such a variety of foods. Oil is technically not included in any of the colors when referring to food but very necessary to add to make a diet filling and nutritious.

Beginning years ago, one of the most unfounded diet recommendations was to go fat-free. I think that Americans have only gotten fatter since then! We need fat in our diets. We need the healthy fats in our diets like olive oil, avocado oil, coconut oil, fish oil and oils found in nuts and avocados. Fat has a myriad number of health benefits. Doctors are now admitting that the medical advice to cut out fat was absolutely wrong. You can look up many YouTube videos showing how detrimental it was to remove healthy fats from our diet. Fats are necessary for many of the body's functions, especially the brain. So add the healthy fats. Stick to avocados, olive oil, avocado oil, coconut oil, real butter and nuts and seeds. Use your judgment as to how much you need a day. So how did I make my food delicious? By adding a modest amount of fat.

The lack of fat in my diet probably set me up for bingeing. I never felt satisfied. My food did not taste good. Fat makes food taste much, much better. Fat helps you feel full. Even a teaspoon or two makes a big difference in your satiation. My cooking is so simple. I usually use some healthy fat, I sprinkle some spices on whatever it is I am cooking and that's it! I now enjoy simply cooked foods that do not have rich sauces. I find them too heavy now. My taste buds have changed, not overnight, but after awhile I started appreciating the taste of real food, not foods altered by being drowned or fried in fat.

You need to figure out which foods make your taste buds sing! So make sure that you try new recipes because being satisfied and enjoying your food also means variety. Do not let boredom set in. Of course, I do have my mainstays; several meals that I rotate often because I truly enjoy them. But it is a good idea to try a new recipe, switch out the same cantaloupe for a new type of melon, or a different spice on your vegetables next time you eat them. Experiment with different vinegars. I love apple cider vinegar and balsamic. I completely replaced sugar in my coleslaw recipes with brown rice vinegar. Did you know brown rice vinegar is sweet? It's delicious! Substitute brown rice vinegar for sugar the next time you make any salad dressing or coleslaw.

You need to figure out what *you* love to eat. Then you can design a menu that incorporates your personal preferences. It might be wise to sit down with a nutritionist or go on-line and search for foods plans. Perusing recipes on different websites will give you ideas of how to go about choosing the foods you love to eat. Keep it simple, though. If you become overwhelmed, you may give up. So try to eat foods that are easy to prepare, yet, really make you happy. Keep it exciting and keep it fun!

Now I know what you may be thinking when I say I truly enjoy eating fruits and vegetables for my snacks. But is there ever room for an occasional piece of cake, donut or pizza?

Yes, there is. The good news is that slim people eat fattening food! However, they eat them infrequently and in controlled portions. They know they are going to eat it again, so they don't have to eat the whole box or bag or a huge amount.

A huge change for my success was to, "Never say never." But rather say "Yes," once in awhile.

Working on my issues eliminated cravings for unhealthy food almost 100% of the time. When I do occasionally decide to eat, let's say, a piece of cake, it is never your typical "junk food." I make sure to eat the highest quality of that particular food possible. Maybe twice a year my husband will look at me at the end of a meal in a restaurant and say, "Want to share a dessert?" I'll say, "Sure," because I know the desserts in that restaurant are amazing and made from real ingredients. I take a few bites and enjoy them with my cup of tea.

Eating clean, real food most of the time has completely changed my taste buds. I can't get over how artificial store bought birthday cake tastes to me now. I can't believe how apparent the taste of artery-clogging margarine is. You couldn't pay me today to eat that garbage. I'm calling it what it is. I ate so much of the artificial, cheap ingredient cakes, cookies and muffins that I had completely messed up my taste buds.

On the chance of sounding really corny, I will tell you that fruit now explodes with flavor in my mouth. I truly enjoy a ripe piece of delicious fruit more than most cakes.

The more I ate clean food, the more I cleaned my palette. The more I cleaned my palette, the more delicious real food tasted. The more delicious my food tasted, the easier I was satisfied and, therefore, the less I needed to eat.

Eat smaller portions, eat clean food and enjoy every delicious bite. While changing your food, make small sustainable changes rather than huge unattainable ones.

Chapter
~ 8 ~

"Write Your Own Story"

1. Are you eating real food?

2. Do you need to clean a fridge and pantry makeover?

3. How does your food need to change? Is organic available? Can you request it where you live?

4. Journal on the importance of eating real food and how it will impact your life.

5. How will you manage to eat smaller portions?

6. How can you make sure to enjoy all the food you eat?

Chapter
~ 9 ~

Maintenance

~ Think, Eat, Drink and Stay Slim ~

I was finally able to maintain my weight when I sustained the changes I made on the levels of mind, body and soul.

For decades I was great at losing weight. I got all hyped up about a new diet. I was perfect for days, weeks, maybe even months. I was so perfect that I even rejected social opportunities to make sure I wasn't tempted to go off my diet. When a very close friends' child was getting married, and I had to go, I packed my dinner and ate it out of a plastic container with a plastic fork in a stairwell of the wedding hall. I was obsessed. I would get to goal, and then what did I do?

I "rewarded" myself by reintroducing all the foods I gave up to lose weight. "I can afford to eat that now," I told myself. My old habits would start creeping back. I would forget to weigh myself. The salads, steamed vegetables, and lean protein started to be replaced with the foods I ate before I went on the most recent diet. I ignored the snug skirt, blaming it on shrinking at the dry cleaners.

Before I knew it, not only did I gain back the weight I lost, but inevitably I weighed even more than I did before. I did this over and over, all the while wallowing in misery, wondering how this happened to me again. How did I gain back all this weight?

Was I insane? The definition of insanity is doing the same thing over and over again and expecting different results. But that is exactly what I kept doing – I slacked off, allowing old behaviors that did not serve me to come back into my life.

The simple truth is that maintaining weight loss requires efforts similar to that of weight loss. I needed to continually reinforce a mindset that supported maintaining my weight loss. Constant mental reminders were necessary to sustain my new habits and to stay on track. I did this by flooding my brain with messages such as:

~ I am slim and healthy.
~ I know how to maintain my weight loss.
~ I can easily maintain my weight loss.
~ I only eat to nourish myself.
~ I am in control; not the food.
~ Will what I am about to eat take me closer to or further away from my goal.
~ Food will not help any problem.
~ No amount of food will fill the voids in my life.
~ I am valuable.
~ I am worth taking care of.
~ Nothing will prevent me from maintaining my goal.
~ No one will prevent me from maintaining my goal.
~ I love myself.

The more I say these, the more I continue to believe them and the more likely I am to stay on track.

I stopped glamorizing the food I ate that made me fat. Those foods are not good for my heart, my blood sugar, my cholesterol, nor my brain. My attitude remains the same as it was when I was losing the weight, "What can I choose to eat to nourish my body now? Which foods will accomplish this?" It truly all begins with my thoughts.

When my weight was still yo-yoing, I'd fall into some kind of mental slumber. The tailored clothes would somehow disappear into the back of my closet and the elastic waistbands would move forward. Not anymore. Every couple of days I make sure to put on the smallest skirt in my closet. After having been obese for so many years, I still need a reminder that I am no longer overweight! Putting on that small size invites the behaviors necessary to ensure maintenance. Sound silly? Maybe. But that works for me.

I print off inspirational quotes on 4" X 6" photo paper and tape them to the front of my kitchen cabinets. I listen to audios that I have created for clients. The audios range from how to kick the sugar habit to eating slowly. I can safely report that every single struggle a client has, I dealt with in the past. That's why all their audios are perfect for me, too. I experiment and change up what I need to do; I rotate reminders so as not to invite weight gain and misery back into my life. Not worth it! Experiment and find what works best for you.

Keeping my food similar to how I ate when I lost weight was paramount to maintenance success. The choices I make now in my food and portion sizes are very similar to what I ate while I was losing. I eat enough to never get too hungry. I eat what I choose to eat. I eat what pleases my taste buds, not what someone else tells me to eat.

I only occasionally eat foods that I used to eat on a daily basis. In my fat days, I did not go a day without cheese at several meals every day. Now I can go months without having any cheese at all. Pizza? I can't believe I thought I could not live without pizza. I loved pizza! I still eat pizza. But only once in a great while. As the years go by, the desire for these foods diminishes greatly as the exhilarating feeling of being slim far outweighs their momentary pleasure.
My habits changed. My choices changed. Most of all, my attitude about food changed for good.

I made lists of foods that lower cholesterol, lower blood sugar and those that deliver the most nutrition per serving. I referred to those often to help me decide what to eat. For example, I read that eating cherries reduces inflammation and the risk of gout, are packed with antioxidants, help you sleep, reduce belly fat, have cancer-preventive benefits and more. I asked myself, "Now what health benefits do I get from eating a cookie?"

This exponentially aided in my maintaining my weight loss. Before long, these choices became routine. I was able to finally chuck those lists into the garbage. Why? The bottom line was always the same. I felt great. My weight stayed the same. Having so many health benefits eating real, clean foods became my food of choice.
Maintenance started to become almost effortless. This does not mean I didn't have to pay attention. I still have to be hyper-vigilant and aware when I notice those demons creeping back into my mind. When cookies and cake beckon,

I stop to see what's going on in my life. I take care of business right then and there, not allowing stuff to pile up. My healthier food choices come back into full swing.

I sometimes take out the "big guns" to keep me on track by employing scare tactics. I replay a short video I saved to my computer. It's a cartoon with cancer cells inside the body. The cartoon depicts healthy, vibrant cells ingesting healthy foods. Those cells are energetically running around getting an "A+" for repairing and regenerating the body. Then there are these little cells that are bandaged, limping and walking with canes. These cells ingested sugar. They are completely debilitated and ridden with cancer. "Okay," I tell myself. Healthy cells it is.

I work on keeping balance in all areas of my life. I continue to nourish myself not only on a physical level, but on the emotional and spiritual levels as well.

Enough self-care is my personal main ingredient in keeping my weight stable. I make sure to do something every single day. It may mean taking only a few minutes to do something "just for me." This is my way of filling my "love tank." I need this filled to keep my equanimity. Notice I rely only on myself, not others. Waiting for others to fill me up never worked. It won't work now. I don't set myself up for disappointment any longer.

I remind myself how much happier I am going to my closet and fitting into every single piece of clothing that is hanging there. I don't have to worry if my clothes fit or don't. They always do! I never want to go back to the days of wondering what fits. I never want to go back to those disappointing days of putting on something that got too tight. Is a piece of cake worth being miserable? Even if I stupidly remember eating a box of cookies as enjoyable, would it be worth not being able to zipper my skirt? No! No food in the world would ever be worth jeopardizing my health. None!

I decided to never, ever, eat again to fill anything other than physical hunger. I broke the bad habits. I refuse to eat to calm a stressful moment, to mend a broken heart, to suppress emotions I'd rather not deal with, to relieve stress from a work deadline or fill boredom. Period.

I never allow myself to gain more than a few pounds. I never need the scale to know when this occurs. I know when I've been a bit too generous with my portions and my tummy feels a tiny bit rounder. I get right back on track. I learned to listen and trust my body. I don't play games. I don't wait till my clothes are tight. That would be too much work. That would be much harder to take off. This method works and keeps things simple.

Last, but certainly not least, I still ask G-d for help. When I start experiencing those ten, twenty or even thirty-year old memories of intense cravings for food swirling around in my head, I ask Him to take away the 'crazies' (my keyword for once again having insane thoughts about desiring foods I know are not good for me). This method has worked, it is working and I know it will work forever.

I am maintaining my weight loss now for more than twenty years. If I can maintain my weight loss, so can you. You can do it!

Chapter
~ 9 ~

"Write Your Own Story"

1. How can you keep maintenance first and foremost in your mind?

2. How can you remember, "I want to be slim and healthy more than anything in the world?"

3. Devise a food plan you can live with the rest of your life.

4. Write down the fattening foods you think you can't live without, and for now, try to reduce the frequency of eating them. Try not eating that food for a week, a month, and so on.

5. How can you keep your "love tank" filled?

6. How can you keep up the positive mindset to always choose nutritious foods?

7. What positive messages/thoughts will you post to keep you motivated?

8. How will you maintain when you reach your goal?

Chapter
~ 10 ~

Time to Write Your Own Story

~ Compilation of End-of-Chapter Notes ~

Now it's time to write your own story.

Refer back to "Write Your Own Story" at the end of Chapters 1 – 9. Read your answers to the questions. Take time for introspection. Think deeply and carefully. Use those answers to create your own holistic plan addressing mind, body and soul.

Be specific and all-encompassing. Leave no stone unturned. Pay special attention to the areas you choose to omit, the ones that are most uncomfortable. Those probably need the most observation.

Make sure your plan addresses questions such as:

Did I contemplate all the areas I need to change in my life?

Which changes will have the biggest impact?

What have I learned that I did not know before? Which changes do I believe I can make that will help me?

What can't I follow exactly but tweak to make it work for me?

What fits into my lifestyle?

Where was I insane?

What mistakes did I repeat?

Which foods am I willing to give up completely?

Which foods will I stop glamorizing?

Which new foods will I try?

Where will I go for support?

The more thorough you are here, the more likely you will cover what needs to be taken care of. Give yourself this gift! But, pace yourself. Change what you know you can maintain.

Set yourself up for success. Focus on changes that will make you a winner. If you know you can't join a gym for financial reasons, don't open a gym membership. Go to a sports equipment store and buy one set of weights. Search YouTube for free workout videos – there are tons! Change what will make you feel great because you accomplished what you set out to do.

If you made a commitment that you could not keep, try another idea. Consider something more in line with what you are already doing, instead of making drastic changes. Major overhauls are rarely successful. Make small, manageable ones. If you have never exercised, try ten or fifteen minutes. Scheduling an hour may lead to exhaustion and soreness. Success breeds success, and helps to keep a positive mindset. A positive mindset is your first-line ammunition in creating positive actions.

Eating out at restaurants five nights a week? Try cutting back to two or three nights. Home cooked food will inevitably be less caloric. No matter how well we order our food in a restaurant, with the best instructions like, "Light on the oil and salt. Dry-grill my chicken, please," we still have more control at home over the salt, oil and portion sizes. The mouth-watering food other diners are eating and the dessert display are also out of sight at home.

Be creative and do not be afraid to try new tactics. Just because something didn't work for you in the past, does not mean it won't work for you now. If something stops working, look for alternatives that will work now. Be flexible and open to making adjustments as your needs change. When your weight loss slows down, change your food and your exercise routine.

What good is it to lament, "I eat the same as my friend and she does cardio only three days a week and I do cardio five days a week - the weight is falling off her and I can't seem to lose a pound!"
Cardio alone may not be your answer. Your genes may respond to a mix of weight training and cardio. You are a unique, amazing individual with your own set of genes that program you in a specific way. Also, learn to examine the whole picture. Do you have more stress in your life? Do you

get enough sleep? It's possible that just improving these two areas will get the scale moving for you, too.

Try anything. Try everything. Nobody gets to the top of a mountain successfully by following an instruction manual. Each toe-hold on the edge of rock has a slightly different angle than the guy before him that made it to the top. The same with weight loss. You need to keep adjusting. You need to look at your final destination to keep up your motivation and to reach your goal.

Never stop trying. Never stop tweaking. Never stop building confidence. Never give up. Never! Explore every single avenue.

It's time for your story to be a story of success, transporting you to a new, beautiful life filled with blessings, happiness, and a slimmer self.

Chapter
~ 10 ~

"Write Your Own Story"

Write *your* story here; your goals, your steps, your food

plan, and the changes you will make on the levels of

body, mind and soul.

About the Author

Rivka Fuchs, AAPC, CMCC, is a Certified Life Coach and Certified Master Coach and Counselor. She is certified in America and in Israel through Refuah Institute.

Coaching is available in person and by phone.
She can be reached by email: rivkafuchscoach@gmail.com

She is passionate about coaching her clients to reach their unique goals.

She is also an artist. Her art can be viewed on Instagram: rivka_fuchs_art

She enjoys her family, friends and clients. She also enjoys being an active community member, volunteering in her spare time.

Acknowledgments

I had typed many random notes on my computer recording my weight-loss successes to keep myself motivated and for reference when my resolve weakened or my memory failed. But writing a book?

I can't say it never occurred to me, but the thought of the whole process was too daunting.

While attending The Institute for Integrative Nutrition, I learned that the founder, Joshua Rosenthal, also offered a book writing course. Which got me thinking. Seriously.

I discussed the slight chance of taking Joshua's "Launch Your Dream Book" course with some friends, and they strongly encouraged me to do so.

Sheri Gumina, www.buildahealthieru.com, and Sarah Christian, www.365lemons.com; how can I thank you enough? Sarah, I still have your email printed and hanging by my desk, "You need to do this. Your story is incredible and you need to share it with the world." You both were truly the impetus that began this endeavor.

I enrolled in the course and never looked back. Joshua Rosenthal, your words still ring in my head. "Excited, not scared." How many times did I freak out and think of dropping out of the course? How many times did I want to ditch the whole effort because writing the book consumed my whole life, greatly limiting the amount of time I spent with family and friends?

Special thanks for the guidance and support to everyone on the Launch Your Dream Book staff. Lindsey Smith, Sue Brown, Shannon Lagasse, Marissa Leigh, Kathleen DiChiara, Patty Bean, Marissa LaRocca, Marie Ann Mosher and fellow classmates – I could not have done it without you.

I also have to thank everyone at Create Space, Amazon's self-publishing arm, for their incredible assistance. I am sure I asked questions that made them roll their eyes, but everyone remained patient and helpful.

Editing was a group effort - an effort of friends and family. Three editors, each with her own unique skills and imprint, made the final manuscript possible.

Judi Schuster. You were the first to read the manuscript. You corrected my spelling, grammatical errors, typo's and a host of other issues. You also wisely suggested splitting larger chapters into smaller, more manageable ones.
You created a new meaning for the word friendship. It goes like this: A true friend is someone that you may not connect with often enough because of your busy lives. A true friend is someone that makes themselves available *immediately* to read your book, even though they work sixty hours a week. A true friend says she loves the book. You are a true friend.

Celine Feinberg. What can I say? I think my friends are the busiest women in the world. How and when did you have the time to take on this commitment? As if you didn't have enough going on in your life. You wear many hats, but I didn't know editing was one of them! I was a little scared at first, thinking you were using your cooking skills. The book was being pared down, paragraphs discarded completely like vegetable peels, and sentences mixed together like batter ingredients. I wanted to say, "Hey, this is a book, not a recipe!" Needless to say, I had no reason to panic. You are as talented an editor as you are at being an amazing friend.

Yakira Apfel. You agreed to edit my book and I was ecstatic. How could I not be? I knew that the author of the first book you edited was so grateful for your outstanding job that he actually paid you more than the originally agreed upon fee. A few weeks later, you apologized for backing out on editing my book, due to lack of time. I admired your decision. However, I knew that your input would be invaluable. Being my daughter, and visiting my house often - thanks for patiently editing bits and pieces. I was quite surprised that you didn't stop coming, knowing that you'd once again be bombarded with a few more pages each visit... "Yakira, can you just take a look at these few pages?" My favorite youngest child.

Jeremy Apfel. I am so grateful for your time and effort. When you offered to read my book, I had no idea you were an expert editor. Your corrections, additions and comments blew me away. Are you sure you are in the right profession? I'd hire you any day. And for the record, you gained lots of points. Not that you needed any. You're already the best in my book.

My dearest husband, Irv. Last but certainly not least. You did the grocery, Costco, and Trader Joe shopping, amongst many other errands. Keep up the good work! (That's our private joke.) Seriously, you supported me every step of the way. Almost every time you approached me to talk, I said, "Not now, I'm in the middle of a thought and I'll lose it. Go

away." Okay. I know what you are thinking. "Almost every time?" No, it was *every* time! You were truly a sport.
But much more importantly, I have to thank you for never, ever saying one word about my weight. There were times that I weighed as much as fifty pounds more than you and you are almost a foot taller than me. Gratitude just doesn't even begin to cut it. You are truly a special guy. Or you need eyeglasses.

Most of all, I know this was all divinely orchestrated. Thank you G-d for squeezing out all that You know I can produce. I pray that I am fulfilling my purpose in this world.

www.ingramcontent.com/pod-product-compliance
Lightning Source LLC
Chambersburg PA
CBHW060905280326
41934CB00007B/1199